The
Complete
Guide
to Lymph
Drainage
Massage

SECOND EDITION

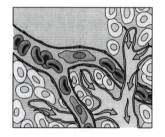

Ramona Moody French

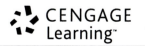

CENGAGE
Learning™

Australia • Canada • Mexico • Singapore • Spain • United Kingdom • United States

![Cengage Learning]

The Complete Guide to Lymph Drainage Massage, Second Edition
Ramona Moody French

President, Editorial: Dawn Gerrain

Acquisitions Editor: Martine Edwards

Product Manager: Danielle Klahr

Editorial Assistant: Sarah Prediletto

Director of Beauty Industry Relations:
 Sandra Bruce

Executive Marketing Manager:
 Gerard McAvey

Associate Marketing Manager: Matthew
 McGuire

Senior Production Director: Wendy Troeger

Senior Art Director: Benjamin Gleeksman

Content Project Management: PreMediaGlobal

For product information and technology assistance, contact us at
Cengage Learning Customer & Sales Support, 1-800-354-9706

For permission to use material from this text or product,
submit all requests online at **www.cengage.com/permissions**
Further permissions questions can be emailed to
permissionrequest@cengage.com

Library of Congress Control Number: 2011938101

ISBN-13: 978-1-4390-5671-4

ISBN-10: 1-4390-5671-4

Milady
Executive Woods
5 Maxwell Drive
Clifton Park, NY 12065
USA

Cengage Learning is a leading provider of customized learning solutions with office locations around the globe, including Singapore, the United Kingdom, Australia, Mexico, Brazil, and Japan. Locate your local office at **www.cengage.com/global**

Cengage Learning products are represented in Canada by Nelson Education, Ltd.

To learn more about Milady, visit **milady.cengage.com**

Purchase any of our products at your local college store or at our preferred online store **www.cengagebrain.com**

Notice to the Reader

Publisher does not warrant or guarantee any of the products described herein or perform any independent analysis in connection with any of the product information contained herein. Publisher does not assume, and expressly disclaims, any obligation to obtain and include information other than that provided to it by the manufacturer. The reader is expressly warned to consider and adopt all safety precautions that might be indicated by the activities described herein and to avoid all potential hazards. By following the instructions contained herein, the reader willingly assumes all risks in connection with such instructions. The publisher makes no representations or warranties of any kind, including but not limited to, the warranties of fitness for particular purpose or merchantability, nor are any such representations implied with respect to the material set forth herein, and the publisher takes no responsibility with respect to such material. The publisher shall not be liable for any special, consequential, or exemplary damages resulting, in whole or part, from the readers' use of, or reliance upon, this material.

Printed in the United States of America
2 3 4 5 6   21 20 19 18 17

To my mentor, Judy Dean.
1933–2003

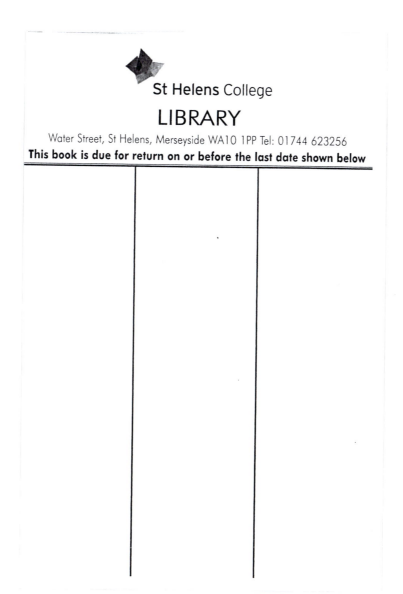

CONTENTS

Preface .... *xi*
About the Author .... *xiv*

CHAPTER 1   THE BIG PICTURE 1
Brief History 2
Understanding Lymph Drainage Massage 2
Understanding Edema 4
Understanding Lymph Diseases 4
   Primary Lymphedema 4
   Secondary Lymphedema 5
Knowing Lymphedema's Effects 5
Working with Lymphedema 5
Review Questions 6

CHAPTER 2   TISSUES AND ORGANS OF THE LYMPHATIC SYSTEM 7
Tissues 8
   Epithelial Tissue 8
   Connective Tissue 9
   Muscle Cells 11
   Nerve Cells 11
   Blood and Lymph 12
Integrated Functions of Organ Systems 13
The Lymphatic System 14
   Lymph 14
   Lymph Vessels 15
   Lymph Nodes 18
Lymph Organs 21
Review Questions 22

CHAPTER 3   LYMPH CIRCULATION 23
Initial Lymphatics 24
Other Factors That Drive Lymph Circulation 24
   The Lymphatic Pump 25
Lymph Drainage Pathways 26
Review Questions 27

CHAPTER 4 FUNCTIONS OF THE LYMPHATIC SYSTEM 28

Immunity 29

Maintain Blood Pressure, Blood Volume, and Fluid
    Balance 29

Preventing Protein Buildup in Tissues 29

Distributing Dietary Fat 30

Healing Injuries 30

New Areas of Research 30

Review Questions 31

CHAPTER 5 IMMUNITY 32

Nonspecific Immunity 33

    Mechanical Methods of Resistance 33

    Chemical Resistance 33

Inflammation 33

Specific Immunity 34

Acquired Immunity 35

Categorizing Cells 35

    Neutrophils 36

    Monocytes and Macrophages 36

    Basophils 36

    Eosinophils 36

    Natural Killer Cells 36

    B- and T-lymphocytes 36

Review Questions 37

CHAPTER 6 EDEMA 38

Understanding Edema Basics 39

    Lack of Exercise 39

    Excessive Dietary Salt 40

    Scar Tissue and Soft Tissue Injury 40

    Heart or Kidney Disease 40

    Medication 40

    Radiation Therapy 40

    Allergies 41

    Menstrual Cycle 41

    Emotional Tension 41

Lymphedema Disease 41

    Primary Lymphedema 43

    Secondary Lymphedema 43

    Working with Lymphedema 43

    Stages of Lymphedema Disease 44

Review Questions 44

**CHAPTER 7 LYMPH DRAINAGE MASSAGE: INDICATIONS
AND CONTRAINDICATIONS** 45

Indications 46

More Indications for LDM 46

    Edema 46

    Surgery 47

    Soft Tissue Injury 47

Sluggish Immune System 47
Relieving Stress and Tension 47
Fatigue, Mild Depression, and Chronic Soft
   Tissue Pain 48
Working with Positional Edema 48
Diet 48
Scar Tissue 48
Enhancing the Skin 49
Contraindications 49
Thrombosis and Phlebitis 49
Risk Factors for Blood Clot (Embolism) 50
Serious Illness 50
Acute Conditions and Infectious Conditions 51
Asthma 51
Allergies 51
Thyroid 51
Low Blood Pressure 51
Intake form 52
Medications (check all that apply) 52
Musculoskeletal symptoms (check all that apply) 52
Skin conditions (check all that apply) 52
Cardiovascular disease (check all
   that apply) 53
Other (check all that apply) 53
Neurological conditions (check all that apply) 53
More 53
Site Restrictions 53
Pressure Restrictions 54
Position Restriction 54
Cancer 54
Pain 54
Activities 55

CHAPTER 8   PRINCIPLES OF LYMPH DRAINAGE MASSAGE 56
Lymph Drainage Massage Principles 57
Palpation 57
Move the Skin 58
Apply Gentle Pressure 58
Move Slowly 59
Direction 59
Rhythm and Repetition 59
Lymph Drainage Patterns 60
Quadrants 61
Executing Face and Neck Patterns 61
Identifying Watersheds 61
Massage Sequence 63
Massage Movements 64
Stationary Circle 64
Pump 64
"J" Strokes 64
Effleurage 65
Review Questions 66

CHAPTER 9   THE LYMPH DRAINAGE MASSAGE SESSION 68

Communication 69

Intake Interview or Consultation 70

Clients' Records Should Include the Following
Information: 70

Preparing for the Massage Session 70

Music 70

The Other Senses 71

Before Beginning The Session 71

Beginning the Session 72

Recording Client Information 72

Activities 73

CHAPTER 10   FACE AND NECK TREATMENT SEQUENCE 74

Indications and Contraindications 75

Swollen Lymph Nodes 76

Locating Lymph Nodes on the Face and Neck 77

Observing and Palpating Lymph Nodes on the Face
and Neck 81

Lymph Drainage Pathways on the Face and Neck 82

Massage Outline 83

Massaging the Neck 84

Massaging the Head 85

CHAPTER 11   LYMPH DRAINAGE MASSAGE OF THE UPPER EXTREMITIES
AND TRUNK 91

Indications 92

Locating Axillary and Breast Lymph Nodes 92

Massage of the Upper Extremity and Trunk 95

Detailed Massage Outline 96

CHAPTER 12   LYMPH DRAINAGE MASSAGE ON THE LOWER EXTREMITIES
AND TRUNK 103

Indications and Contraindications 104

Locating Inguinal Lymph Nodes 104

Observing and Palpating the Inguinal Lymph Nodes 106

Massage Procedure: Massaging the Inguinal Nodes,
Abdomen and Affected Leg 107

Step-by-Step: Massaging the Inguinal Nodes, Abdomen,
and Affected Leg 108

Massaging the Affected Lower Limb 109

CHAPTER 13   ABDOMINAL MASSAGE: STIMULATING THE DEEP
CIRCULATION OF LYMPH 116

Contraindications 118

Structure 118

Skeletal Structure 119

Lower Ribs 120

Lumbar Spine 120

Ilium 120

Pubis Symphysis and Pubic Ridge 122

Inguinal Ligament 122
Organs 122
    Abdominal Aorta 122
    Stomach. 122
    Spleen 122
    Liver and Gallbladder 122
    Small Intestine. 123
    Bladder 124
    Reproductive Organs 124
Muscles and Fascia 124
    Rectus Abdominis 124
    External Oblique 124
    Internal Oblique 124
    Transversus Abdominis 124
    Diaphragm 125
    Psoas Major. 125
    Iliacus 125
    Quadratus Lumborum 125
    Piriformis 126
    Levator Ani 126
Fascia. 126
Nodes and Vessels 127
    Outline of Abdominal Massage 132
    Massage the Superficial Muscles and Connective
        Tissue 132
    Stretch the Deeper Connective Tissue 134
    Locate Deeper Muscles 134
    Pumping the Cisterna Chyli 135
Notes 135

CHAPTER 14 ENERGETIC AND MIND-BODY EFFECTS OF LYMPH
DRAINAGE MASSAGE 136
Establishing the Proper Setting 137
The Meditative Touch. 137
Preparing the Client. 138
Healing Crisis 140
    Understanding the Health Crisis 140
    Dangers of Emotional Release Work 141
    Other Problems from Emotional Release Work:
        Interpretation 143
    Identification 143
    Enmeshment 143
    Judgment 143
    People-pleaser 143
    Boundaries 144
Review Questions 144

CHAPTER 15 USING LYMPH DRAINAGE MASSAGE
WITH OTHER TREATMENTS 145
Soft-Tissue Injury. 146
Reducing Fibrosis and Scar Tissue. 147

Complementing Skin Care 148
Body-Mind Therapies. 148
Detoxification treatments 148
Cellulite 150
Introducing Cellulite 150
Remedying Cellulite 151
Treating the Body. 151
Outline of Cellulite Massage 152
Connective tissue massage. 153
Lymph drainage massage 154

CHAPTER 16 **SELF-MASSAGE USING LYMPH DRAINAGE**
MASSAGE TECHNIQUES 156
Self-Massaging the Face and Neck. 158
Step-by-Step: Focusing on the Neck. 159
Step-by-Step: Massaging the Face 160
Step-by-Step: Self-Massage of the Upper Limbs. 164
Step-by-Step: Self-Massaging the Lower Limbs 169
Treating Soft-Tissue Injuries 172

CHAPTER 17 **HEALING CRISIS** 173
Understanding the Healing Crisis 174

ANSWER KEY 177
REFERENCES/ENDNOTES 182
GLOSSARY 185
RESOURCES 190
INDEX 191

Although it was described before the blood circulatory system[1] in the seventeenth century, the lymphatic system has been largely ignored and misunderstood. The greatest advances in understanding the lymphatic system came in the twentieth century. More attention, and therefore more research, has been focused on the immune system, of which the lymphatic system is a large part. Research into lymphology has increased modern understanding of the lymphatic system, and it has increased the understanding of, and treatment for, lymphedema disease.

While the term *lymph drainage* was evidently coined by Frederic P. Millard,[2] an osteopath in Ontario, Canada, modern LDM was developed by Drs. Emil and Estrid Vodder in France in the 1930s. Dr. Emil Vodder originally developed the technique to treat sinus infections, enlarged lymph nodes, and acne. He realized that it could play an important part in improving the appearance of healthy people and announced his technique to the cosmetology industry in France. LDM quickly became an important technique for the beauty industry.

Lymphology research and oncology research are related, because lymphedema disease is often a result of cancer treatment. For decades, however, little help was offered during follow-up treatment for cancer patients suffering painful and disfiguring lymphedema disease. Today, there is a greater awareness of lymphedema disease among doctors and the public, in part, because patients have tried to understand and seek help for this condition. Many self-help groups for lymphedema patients have formed, and national groups like the National Lymphedema Network[3] serve patients, therapists, and physicians by disseminating information about lymphedema disease and its treatment.

Many professionals today, including physical therapists, nurses, massage therapists, and estheticians, use LDM techniques. This book is for massage therapists, estheticians, nurses, and others who use massage as part of their work. It also helps patients with edema or lymphedema to understand the lymphatic system and possibly learn how to perform LDM on themselves.

Lymph drainage massage is used widely in esthetics/cosmetology because it improves the skin's appearance. The focus of esthetics is beauty, but it has always included health, because beauty really does come from the inside, and health definitely affects appearance. Esthetics journals frequently offer information on LDM's techniques and cosmetology applications. The manufacturers and distributors of cosmetology products offer LDM training. While very effective, the disadvantage of this training is that it may fail to include a great deal of information on contraindications and safety. LDM has important beneficial physiological effects on the body, but it is not appropriate or even safe for everyone.

Massage therapists long viewed LDM as a specialty involving expensive training in foreign locations, and perceived it mainly as medical massage for lymphedema treatment. When I began massage training, LDM was not regularly offered at any massage school of which I was aware, and it was difficult to find LDM teachers. Now, however, massage therapists have discovered that LDM not only benefits lymphedema and beauty treatments, it is an effective tool for body-mind work, stress reduction, and soft-tissue pain reduction. LDM is used in sports massage, which was the first kind of massage to become mainstream, in the 1980s. Also, LDM is deeply meditative and, in the right setting, produces an altered state of consciousness in both therapist and client.

There are now more schools of thought about how LDM should be performed. The Vodder method of LDM is perhaps the most widely known, but since the 1930s, others have researched and experimented with various techniques to move fluid out of soft tissues and into the bloodstream. Lymphology is an unusual field in that there is organized communication and support between medical practitioners and researchers, massage therapists, and patients.

Modern LDM techniques are often simple and easy to learn, and just as effective as more time-honored systems. Self-massage methods help patients who lack access to professional therapists or who cannot afford daily professional therapy, which can be both expensive and time-consuming. Massage therapists and estheticians have different but overlapping scopes of practice. Because I am a massage therapist, I may mention massage therapists more often than estheticians in this text, but the information applies to both fields. I based this text on material I have used in the classroom over the past 28 years as a practitioner and teacher of massage, especially LDM. This material is meant to be simple for beginning lymph drainage massage therapists to use and understand. I wanted a book that explains, in ordinary language, the structure, circulation, and function of the lymphatic system and the indications and contraindications for LDM.

I wanted to write a text that makes basic lymphatic system information accessible and understandable for a wide variety of students. I also wanted to create a minimalist approach to LDM that, despite its simplicity, still very effectively moves fluid through the lymphatic system. After years of experimenting in my practice and in the classroom, I have devised such a technique, one that therapists and their clients can use for various needs and situations. Medical research supports the idea that very simple techniques can increase lymph uptake and movement through the lymphatic system.[4]

In addition to showing me the merits of simplicity, my experience has taught me that massage therapists and estheticians need not learn everything about the lymphatic system and LDM before working on clients, especially in a wellness practice. What is important is that practitioners learn the massage technique well, and that they understand the indications and contraindications for LDM. It is crucial that therapists and estheticians practice LDM as they continue training. Many who are not seriously ill can benefit from skilled LDM, and therapists can safely work on these clients while continuing to refine their knowledge and palpation skills. The more clients that therapists work on, the more the therapists' sensitivity, palpation skills, and technique improve. As they develop their knowledge and tactile skills, LDM therapists should continue to study and take LDM courses.

I am very grateful to my friends Mariellen and Burt Boss, excellent lymph drainage massage therapists with whom I worked for years. I appreciate the wonderful staff at Milady/Cengage who produced this book, especially Maria Hebert, Philip Mandl and Martine Edwards. Thank you very much! I learned a lot about touch in general and lymph drainage massage specifically from my mentors, two guiding lights in the massage profession who have now passed on: Judy Dean and E.W. Mueller, of Mueller College in San Diego.

I have been a massage therapist for 29 years. My first exposure to lymph drainage massage (LDM) was in a workshop taught by a colleague. I began to use LDM techniques in my practice and to look for other teachers so I could learn more techniques for reducing swelling, whether they were called LDM or not.

In addition to seeking more training and practice, I began systematically surveying the medical literature to learn more about the lymphatic system and lymph drainage massage. Because LDM is the most scientifically researched style of massage, a great deal of information is available.

During study trips to China, I was very interested to observe how *tui na* massage techniques were used to reduce edema in injuries, and I began to add these techniques to my LDM practice. It was interesting to see that *tui na* practitioners patiently repeat the same stationary circle very slowly until they can feel a change in the tissue, and work from the periphery of a swelling toward the center over time. These medical doctors explained *tui na* techniques in terms of traditional Chinese medicine rather than the lymphatic system. The techniques used by these doctors effectively reduce edema, whatever the explanation or theory behind their use.

Since my first LDM exposure, I have experimented with techniques based on what I read in medical journals and other sources, letting what I learned shape my practice. Information about the lymphatic system has exploded in the last century, and the field of lymphology is expanding. New information, as it develops, will contribute to changes in techniques and practitioners' understanding of how massage affects the lymphatic system, and thereby human physiology and health. Such material has shaped my LDM experimentation and has inspired the conclusions in this text.

Over the years, LDM became a form of movement meditation for me. Success depends as much on being mindful and present as on technique. I found I was not only helping my clients, I was helping myself. Through LDM, I gained the benefits usually ascribed to meditation. I became more relaxed and peaceful, more mindful and centered in all activities, better able to deal with stress. One of LDM's many benefits is its positive effect on the therapist. For me, LDM is a form of meditation, with all its attendant effects on life and living. Lymph drainage massage becomes more a matter of "being" than "doing."

The Big Picture

Lymph drainage massage (LDM), a gentle, rhythmic style of massage that mimics the action of the **lymphatic system**, uses precise rhythm and pressure to open the initial lymphatics and stimulate lymph vessel contraction to reduce **edema**. Edema is an unusual accumulation of fluid in soft tissues that can be temporary and mild, or serious, as in chronic lymphedema. Lymph massage strokes do not slide over the skin, but press gently into the skin, moving it without increasing blood circulation or reaching the depth of muscle tissue.[1]

BRIEF HISTORY

In the late 19th century, Alexander von Winiwater of Austria developed specialized massage and compression treatments for lymphedema disease. In the 1930s, Emil Vodder, a Danish physiotherapist, and his wife developed a method of massaging the lymph nodes of patients with colds. In 1963, Dr. Johannes Asdonk learned the Vodder massage method and subsequently established a school in Germany with the Vodders as instructors. Eventually, the Vodders moved to Austria to open their own school. Dr. Asdonk founded the German Society of Lymphology in 1976 with Kuhnke, Foldi and others. Since then, manual lymph drainage has been further developed by Leduc, and later by Foldi and Casley-Smith. These scientists developed comprehensive decongestive therapy (CDT), a combination of LDM, bandaging, exercise and skin care that is more effective in the treatment of lymphedema disease than massage alone. [2, 3, 4, 5, 6, 7, 8]

UNDERSTANDING LYMPH DRAINAGE MASSAGE

LDM uses external massage strokes to move fluids out of body tissues and into the lymphatic system. LDM mimics the lymphatic system, employing repetitive strokes at a precise speed, rhythm, and pressure. LDM stimulates the **immune system**, because it helps move stagnant tissue fluid out of tissues and into the **lymphatic vessels**, where it is transported through the **lymph nodes** and purified by **lymphocytes**.

When performing LDM, the therapist moves the client's skin in different directions: lengthwise, horizontally, and diagonally. These movements, which stretch the microfilaments just below the skin that control the openings to the initial lymphatics (the start of the lymph vessels which allow entrance of fluid into the lymphatic system), allow **interstitial fluid** to enter the lymphatic system while stimulating the lymph vessels to contract.[9] Interstitial fluid is the solution that bathes and surrounds the body's cells. Fluids are propelled forward through the lymph vessels and away from tissue areas where fluid has pooled. LDM stimulates the lymphatic vessels to contract more frequently. It also appears to make natural contractions more regular.

In addition to improving fluid flow, LDM is very relaxing. The method's slow, gentle, repetitive movements reduce the body's "fight-or-flight response" to stress (a function of the sympathetic nervous system) and stimulate the body's parasympathetic reaction. The fight-or-flight reaction causes the body to tense and to produce hormones and chemicals for defense. This reaction also depresses the immune system while stressing many body systems, including the cardiovascular system. Over time, such stress can cause physical damage. LDM helps to put the body into a parasympathetic state, which slows the heart rate and breathing, relaxes muscles, and allows organs to resume normal functioning.

Although other massage styles, like Swedish massage, can move tissue fluids, they lack the specificity that is the basis of successful lymph work. LDM is very light, gentle, and strictly paced. It does not use long strokes, heavy pressure, or rapid movements such as percussion. LDM is not painful.

Dr. Vodder focused on using lymph drainage massage to enhance the immune system of relatively healthy people, establishing the importance of LDM in a wellness setting. The focus of the scientists who followed Vodder has been on the treatment of lymphedema disease. So, LDM is important in two areas: enhancing lymph circulation and immunity and maintaining health on the one hand, and the treatment of chronic edema, lymphedema disease, on the other hand. Working with LDM in the wellness setting is different from working with LDM in a clinical setting. Working in wellness care would not require every client to be medically supervised.

In the wellness setting, LDM is used to enhance lymph circulation and the distribution of leukocytes throughout the body, which enhances the immune system. It is used to reduce pain and edema, and improve the appearance and health of the skin. LDM is deeply relaxing and can be used when massaging clients with high stress levels. Because LDM is so relaxing, it is a useful technique for body-mind work. LDM can be combined with sports massage, deep tissue massage and body treatment in cases of disease or injury. It helps to speed healing of injuries, and reduce scar tissue, so it is beneficial for sports injuries.

In a clinical setting, LDM is used after cosmetic surgery to reduce swelling, speed healing and reduce the development of scar tissue. It is used in the treatment of lymphedema disease, which is chronic obstructive edema that can develop after surgery, injury or radiation treatment. It is part of comprehensive decongestive therapy, along with non-elastic bandages, compression garments, exercise and skin care. Bandaging and exercise for lymphedema disease are not covered in this text; instead, the focus is solely on lymph drainage massage.

Lymph drainage helps to reduce scar tissue. Scar tissue responds slowly to massage and repeated sessions are required to obtain visible results. Progress is faster if LDM is combined with connective tissue massage, such as skin rolling or cross-fiber friction.

LDM helps speed healing of injuries by stimulating microcirculation, which assists in the removal of cellular debris from the site of the injury. As the lymphatic system removes toxins and damaged cells, increased blood flow brings nutrients and fibers that will be used to repair injured tissues. Massaging as soon as safe after an injury minimizes the amount of scar tissue that forms, and improves tissue structure.

Even old scars can benefit from LDM, which can help scars to become softer, smoother, and more flexible. Progress is slow, however, so it is a good idea to teach clients to self-treat daily. A combination of connective tissue massage, such as deep-tissue massage or myofascial release with LDM, produces the best results.

Something for massage therapists and estheticians to understand is that there is a difference between the techniques we use, the results that we believe can be attributed to those techniques, and our beliefs about why we get those results. Scientific research has shown that some of the things we used to believe about the effects of lymph drainage massage aren't true, and has validated other beliefs. Rather than continuing to repeat traditional ideas about the effects of LDM, we should stay informed about current scientific research so that we can be accurate when speaking about our work to our clients.

How can massage therapists, estheticians and other caregivers stay informed about scientific progress in the field of lymph drainage massage? Subscribe to professional journals such as "Lymphology," use online resources to research answers to your client's questions and continue to take classes in lymph drainage massage. Attend conferences where you can talk with other professionals, sharing information and experiences.

UNDERSTANDING EDEMA

Edema is a condition in which excess interstitial fluid saturates tissues, causing them to swell. Edema means that lymphatic flow in that area is overloaded.[10]

Edema can be a temporary problem due to a variety of factors, such as too much salt in the diet, which causes fluid retention. Muscle contraction and relaxation and low-amplitude body movements stimulate lymph circulation. Therefore, a sedentary lifestyle can lead to edema because there is too little activity to stimulate lymph circulation. Tissue fluids also respond to gravity, so inactivity can cause these fluids to pool in the legs, ankles, and lower areas of the body. The legs and ankles can also hold too much fluid in cases of a weak heart, kidney failure, hypothyroidism, and other hormonal imbalances. In addition, edema can result from such minor injuries as contusions or burns as part of the inflammatory response. Scar tissue can also block lymphatic circulation, causing edema.

Edema may also occur over tissues that are stiff due to emotional trauma. Stress and the fight-or-flight response cause muscles to tighten and to remain tight. Massage therapists, estheticians, and others who perform LDM often observe that their clients possess this combination of tissue conditions, chronic muscle stiffness, and **lymph stasis** due to stress. This combination can be seen most clearly over thigh and hip muscles, and shoulder and neck muscles.

UNDERSTANDING LYMPH DISEASES

Primary Lymphedema

Primary lymphedema is due to the congenital malformation of blood and/or lymph vessels. For instance, there may be an abnormal abundance of blood vessels in one leg. In that case, the surplus blood vessels would release more tissue fluids into the tissues of the leg than the lymphatic system could absorb and carry away from the limb. This would cause chronic edema in the affected leg, while the other limb remained normal. In another case, the cause of congenital lymphedema is a lack of lymph vessels in an area because the lymphatic system did not develop properly before birth. More women than men experience congenital lymphedema disease.

Secondary Lymphedema

Secondary lymphedema is caused by obstruction due to infection, injury, irradiation, or surgery. In Africa, for instance, **elephantiasis** is a very advanced form of lymphedema caused by a parasite that infects and scars the lymphatics. In more developed countries, lymphedema often follows cancer surgery, which often removes tissue, including lymph nodes, and causes scarring. Radiation therapy scars the tissues through which it passes, hardening those tissues as if they had been cooked.

KNOWING LYMPHEDEMA'S EFFECTS

Lymphedema disease has serious complications. Because of scar tissue, fluid is not removed from tissues normally. Instead, the fluid stays in the tissues and stagnates. Bacteria can multiply and cause cellulitis, the painful inflammation of subcutaneous connective tissue. Cellulitis is caused by bacteria entering the skin, and can develop into a serious infection that is difficult to heal and can sometimes lead to amputation. Chronic lymphedema disease can cause the skin to thicken, cool and coarsen and become prone to injury and infection. The body treats proteins in stagnant interstitial fluid as foreign particles, which causes **inflammation** and its symptoms of pain, heat, redness, and more edema. Chronic inflammation creates a sort of feedback loop in which the inflammation causes tissues to scar, and scar tissue blocks lymph circulation. As the capacity of the lymphatic system becomes limited, blood vessels continue to release fluid into those tissues, increasing the edema. This causes stress on the skin and **connective tissue** which causes more inflammation. The gross deformities of elephantiasis show how severe the problem can become.

Patients with lymphedema disease must scrupulously protect their edematous limbs from injury and infection. Chronic lymphedema disease is painful and disfiguring, and patients with lymphedema disease may struggle with depression because the disease limits their ability to move and function normally. A severe case can render a patient housebound and sedentary.

WORKING WITH LYMPHEDEMA

Clearly, working with lymphedema disease is a job for experienced practitioners who have had advanced training and some clinical practice. In clinical practice, under supervision, therapists are more aware of contraindications and the serious problems that might arise in treatment. They gain experience dealing with all the manifestations of lymphedema. Beginning LDM therapists should not be afraid to help anyone who comes to them, but should definitely work under the supervision of an experienced therapist or medical practitioner.

REVIEW QUESTIONS

1. Who is the first doctor who developed a method of lymph drainage massage?
2. Which doctor opened the first school that offered training in lymph drainage massage?
3. What is comprehensive decongestive therapy?
4. What are the effects of LDM?
5. How is LDM performed?
6. What is the purpose of LDM?
7. What are the physiological effects of LDM?
8. What is edema?
9. Compare and contrast LDM for the clinical setting and the wellness setting.
10. What factors can cause edema?.
11. What is primary lymphedema?.
12. What is secondary lymphedema?.
13. What factors or events can cause obstructive lymphedema?
14. Describe some complications of lymphedema.

Tissues and Organs
of the Lymphatic System

T he lymphatic system is an amazing system, intimately connected to all the other systems of the body, working with them to provide **immunity** against disease and remove toxins and metabolic waste. This chapter describes basic information about the organization of the cells, tissues, and organs of the lymphatic system to aid massage therapists and estheticians to understand how massage affects the lymphatic system. This chapter also describes how all the systems of the body work together to provide different forms of immunity.

TISSUES

Tissues are groups of similar cells. The human body is made up of four kinds of tissues: epithelial tissue, connective tissue, muscle tissue, and nervous tissue. Connective tissue provides support and structure. Epithelial tissues cover and line organs and vessels. Muscle tissue includes striated (also called voluntary) muscles that move the skeleton, and smooth muscle (also called involuntary), such as the muscles that form the walls of blood and lymph vessels. Nerve tissue is made up of nerve cells (neurons) and is used to carry messages between the brain and the rest of the body.

In addition to those four tissues, there are various fluids in the body such as blood, lymph and tissue fluid. Fluids pass through all the membranes of the body, carrying nutrients and white blood cells to all the tissues of the body and carrying waste away from tissue cells.

The space outside of tissue cells is called the extracellular or **interstitial space**. This space is filled with a substance known as the extracellular matrix or ground substance. Ground substance is a term that describes all of the non-cellular components of the extracellular matrix which contains the fibers that act as a support for cells. It is a gel composed of interstitial fluid (water, inorganic salts, nutrients and waste products), complex sugar molecules and fibrous proteins. Ground substance can be more or less fluid, depending on the area and function. For instance, cartilage is stiffer than other tissues, due to the particular composition of the ground substance.

Epithelial Tissue

Epithelial tissue forms the surfaces and linings of the body, including the skin, the surface of organs, and the lining of the respiratory and digestive tracts. Internal epithelial tissues are called endothelium. Epithelial tissue has a variety of functions. It protects, contains, separates, forms membranes, and contains specialized cells such as sensory nerves in the skin, eyes, ears, nose and tongue.

Epithelial tissue known as glandular epithelial tissue forms endocrine (internal secretion) and exocrine (external secretion) glands that secrete enzymes, hormones, and fluids such as sweat and mucus (Figure 2–1).

Single layer epithelial tissue forms membranes that permit the movement of gases, nutrients, and liquids throughout the body. For instance, **epithelial cells** lining the small intestines permit the passage of dietary nutrients from the intestines to the blood and **lymph vessels**. The walls of blood and lymph vessels are permeable, allowing fluid to circulate from blood vessels to tissue cells to lymphatic vessels (Figure 2–2).

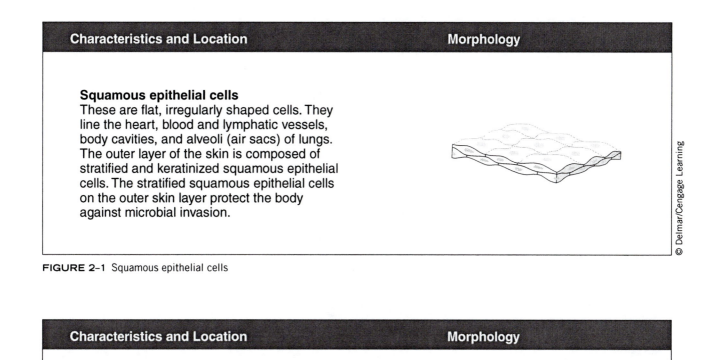

Characteristics and Location	Morphology
Squamous epithelial cells These are flat, irregularly shaped cells. They line the heart, blood and lymphatic vessels, body cavities, and alveoli (air sacs) of lungs. The outer layer of the skin is composed of stratified and keratinized squamous epithelial cells. The stratified squamous epithelial cells on the outer skin layer protect the body against microbial invasion.	

© Delmar/Cengage Learning

FIGURE 2–1 Squamous epithelial cells

Characteristics and Location	Morphology
Columnar epithelial cells Elongated, with the nucleus generally near the bottom and often ciliated on the outer surface; they line the ducts, digestive tract (especially the intestinal and stomach lining), parts of the respiratory tract, and glands.	

© Delmar/Cengage Learning

FIGURE 2–2 Columnar epithelial cells

Connective Tissue

Connective tissue is composed of a variety of types of cells that provide the human body with support, protection, and structure. Connective tissue includes cartilage, tendons, ligaments, fascia, bone, lymph, blood, and fat tissue. Connective tissues contain collagen bundles (inflexible fibers) and elastin (flexible fibers) which are imbedded in a matrix or ground substance, that can be liquid, semisolid, or solid. Blood and lymph are a liquid connective tissue, with less structure than muscles, tendons, or bones. Bone is made of bone cells (osteocytes) surrounded by ground substance that is very hard due to accumulation of minerals (mainly calcium and phosphorus).

The most common kind of connective tissue is loose connective tissue. Loose connective tissue includes **areolar tissue**, **adipose tissue** and **reticular tissue**. Areolar connective tissue wraps around organs, muscles, blood vessels, nerves, spinal cord, and brain. It forms a layer beneath mucus tissues that line all organ systems which are open to the outside of the body. Areolar tissue contains more fluid than other tissues, which makes the distribution of nutrients from blood vessels to muscles and organs possible. Because loose connective

Function	Characteristics and Location	Morphology

Areolar (loose) connective
This tissue surrounds various organs and supports both nerve cells and blood vessels, which transport nutrient material (to cells) and wastes (away from cells). Areolar tissue also (temporarily) stores glucose, salts, and water.

It is composed of a large, semifluid matrix, with many different types of cells and fibers embedded in it. These include fibroblasts (fibrocytes), plasma cells, macrophages, mast cells, and various white blood cells. The fibers are bundles of strong, flexible white fibrous protein called collagen, and elastic single fibers of elastin. It is found in the epidermis of the skin and in the subcutaneous layer with adipose cells.

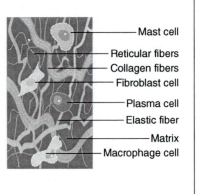

FIGURE 2–3 Areolar tissue

tissue cells are relatively far apart and surrounded by fluid, lymphocytes are able to migrate through areolar connective tissue and attack pathogens that may be present (Figure 2–3).

Reticular connective tissue is a mesh, similar to areolar connective tissue, but is more organized and dense. It forms a scaffold of fibers that supports the **spleen**, red bone marrow and lymph nodes. Adipose tissue is loose connective tissue that contains fat cells (Figure 2–4).

Dense connective tissue is made of fibers that are flexible but not elastic. Dense connective tissue includes strong tissues such as ligaments, tendons, aponeuroses, and fascia. Ligaments are very strong inelastic tissues that support joints (Figure 2–5). Tendons connect muscles to bones, and fascia wraps around

Function	Characteristics and Location	Morphology

Adipose tissue
This tissue stores lipid (fat), acts as filler tissue, cushions, supports, and insulates the body.

A type of loose, connective tissue composed of sac-like adipose cells; they are specialized for the storage of fat. Adipose cells are found throughout the body: in the subcutaneous skin layer, around the kidneys, within padding around joints, and in the marrow of long bones.

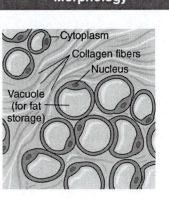

FIGURE 2–4 Adipose tissue

Function	Characteristics and Location	Morphology
Dense fibrous This tissue forms ligaments, tendons, and aponeuroses. **Ligaments** are strong, flexible bands (or cords) that hold bones firmly together at the joints. **Tendons** are white, glistening bands attaching skeletal muscles to the bones. **Aponeuroses** are flat, wide bands of tissue holding one muscle to another or to the periosteum (bone covering). **Fasciae** are fibrous connective tissue sheets that wrap around muscle bundles to hold them in place.	Dense fibrous tissue is also called white fibrous tissue, because it is made from closely packed white collagen fibers. Fibrous tissue is flexible but not elastic. This tissue has a poor blood supply and heals slowly.	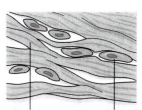 Closely packed collagen fibers Fibroblast cell

© Delmar/Cengage Learning

FIGURE 2–5 Dense connective tissue

muscles cells and individual muscles, as well as muscle groups. Aponeuroses are a form of tendon: broad sheets of very tough connective tissue that hold muscles to each other and to bones.

Cartilage is connective tissue composed of collagen and cells embedded in a gel matrix called chondrin. Hyaline cartilage (contains no visible fibers) cushions the articulations of bones in joints, and connects ribs to the sternum. It is also found in the nose, ears, larynx, and trachea. Fibrocartilage (contains a large amount of collagen fibers visible under the microscope) is found in the intervertebral disks and the pubic symphysis, and is somewhat flexible, allowing for movement. Elastic cartilage is found in the ears (contains large amounts of elastin).

Muscle Cells

Muscle cells have the ability to contract and relax, providing movement in the body. Connective tissue binds the skeletal muscle tissue to the skeleton. When muscle cells contract, the connective tissue pulls on attachment sites on bones, moving the bones closer together. Smooth muscle cells form the muscle layers in the walls of blood and lymph vessels, and the walls of hollow organs such as the stomach and intestines. Cardiac muscle is only found in the heart, and has characteristics of both skeletal muscle fibers and smooth muscle fibers (Figure 2–6).

Nerve Cells

Nerve cells enable sense organs such as the eyes, nose, mouth and nerve cells in the skin to sense stimuli. Nerve impulses are carried to the central nervous system, the brain and spinal cord, where they are interpreted. The central

Function	Characteristics and Location	Morphology
Smooth (nonstriated involuntary) These provide for involuntary movement. Examples include the movement of materials along the digestive tract, controlling the diameter of blood vessels and the pupils of the eyes.	Smooth muscle is nonstriated because it lacks the obvious striations (bands) of skeletal muscles; its movement is involuntary. It makes up the walls of the digestive, genitourinary, and respiratory tracts, blood vessels, and lymphatic vessels.	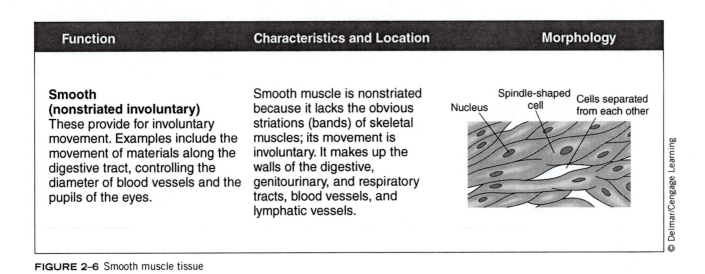

FIGURE 2–6 Smooth muscle tissue

nervous system responds by sending out nerve impulses to muscles, signaling them to respond to the original stimulus. The autonomic nervous system transmits nerve impulses to involuntary muscles and glands.

Blood and Lymph

Blood is a liquid that contains **erythrocytes**, **leukocytes**, and **platelets** (Figure 2–7). Lymph is a liquid that contains leukocytes, protein, and **metabolic waste** (Figure 2–8).

Plasma, interstitial fluid, and lymph are essentially the same liquid matrix, although the contents of the fluid varies according to location and function. Fluid migrates through membranes, including blood and lymph vessels, cell walls

Function	Characteristics and Location	Morphology
Vascular (liquid blood tissue) Blood Transports nutrients and oxygen molecules to cells and metabolic wastes away from cells (can be considered as a liquid tissue). Contains cells that function in the body's defense and in blood clotting.	Blood is composed of two major parts: a liquid called plasma, and a solid cellular portion known as blood cells (or corpuscles). The plasma suspends corpuscles, of which there are two major types: red blood cells (erythrocytes) and white blood cells (leukocytes). A third cellular component (really a cell fragment) is called platelets (thrombocytes). Blood circulates within the blood vessels (arteries, veins, and capillaries) and through the heart.	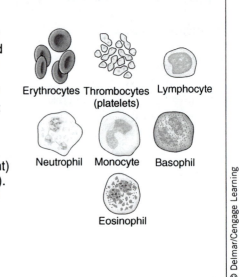

FIGURE 2–7 Blood

Function	Characteristics and Location	Morphology
Lymph Transports tissue fluid, proteins, fats, and other materials from the tissues to the circulatory system. This occurs through a series of tubes called the lymphatic vessels.	Lymph is a fluid made up of water, glucose, protein, fats, and salt. The cellular components are lymphocytes and granulocytes. They flow in tubes called lymphatic vessels, which closely parallel the veins and bathe the tissue spaces between cells.	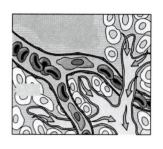

© Delmar/Cengage Learning

FIGURE 2-8 Lymph

and the membranes surrounding muscles, bones and organs. Blood transports oxygen, nutrients and immune cells to all tissues of the body. Interstitial fluid which surrounds blood vessels, lymph vessels, muscles, and organs, supports the distribution of oxygen and nutrients to tissue cells, and the removal of metabolic waste which is then absorbed into the lymphatic system and the cardiovascular system to be eliminated.

Lymph carries **toxins** (microorganisms, microscopic particles, chemicals) and natural products (proteins, and metabolic waste) away from tissues to lymph nodes, where it is purified. Lymph is then propelled through larger and larger lymph vessels until it is returned to the cardiovascular system.

INTEGRATED FUNCTIONS OF ORGAN SYSTEMS

The cardiovascular system distributes immune cells from bone marrow to the entire body. Plasma filters out of blood **capillaries** into tissues, carrying immune cells and nutrients to tissue cells.

The respiratory system stimulates lymph circulation through respiration and exhalation. As the diaphragm moves downward during inhalation, it compresses abdominal organs, causing them to move inferiorly and anteriorly. During exhalation, the diaphragm relaxes and moves upward, causing abdominal organs to move upward as well. This regular movement massages lymph vessels in the **abdomen**, stimulating lymph circulation. During inhalation, the lungs expand and compress the **thoracic duct**, causing it to empty into the subclavian and/or jugular veins. During exhalation, pressure on the thoracic duct relaxes and causes lymph fluid to move into the thoracic duct from abdominal and thoracic lymph trunks.

The epithelial cells lining the respiratory tract have flexible extensions called **cilia**, which are like tiny fingers that roll microscopic foreign particles upward out of the respiratory system. They are coughed up and swallowed, enter into the digestive system, and are destroyed by stomach acid.

The digestive system contains **lymph nodules** which process pathogens that enter the body when food or fluids are ingested. The digestive system also contains **lacteals**, lymph vessels that carry digested dietary fat from the intestines to the thoracic duct. Each organ in the digestive system has its own lymph nodes, which also empty into lymph vessels leading to the thoracic duct. Sufficient digestive acid in the stomach is necessary to destroy microorganisms that are ingested with food.

The muscular system stimulates lymph circulation in two ways: through muscular contraction and relaxation which moves lymph through the muscles themselves, and through skeletal movement which stimulates peripheral lymph circulation by stretching the openings to the initial lymphatics. The walls of the vascular and lymphatic vessels are composed of smooth muscle tissue which expands and contracts involuntarily to aid the movement of fluid containing lymphocytes through the cardiovascular and lymphatic systems.

Smooth muscle cells are found in the walls of hollow organs such as the stomach and intestines, the bladder, the uterus, and the walls of blood and lymph vessels. Smooth muscle cells control involuntary movement such as intestinal peristalsis in the abdomen as well as the **lymphatic pump**, which is the alternate contraction and relaxation of the walls of the **lymphangions**, the functional unit of a lymph vessel and an important part of lymph circulation.

The skeletal system contributes to immunity through the development of immune cells in bone marrow, which are distributed throughout the body by the cardiovascular and lymphatic systems.

The **thymus** is part of the endocrine system. The thymus secretes thymosin, a hormone which signals immune cells to mature into T-cells.

The integumentary system is part of the non-specific immune system. It prevents pathogens, chemical and foreign particles from entering the body, and secretes fluids and chemicals which wash away pathogens, microscopic particles and chemicals that are harmful to the organism, as well as preventing pathogens from multiplying on the surface of the skin. The skin also helps to conserve body fluids.

The autonomic nervous system transmits nerve impulses to involuntary muscles, including the smooth muscle cells forming the muscular walls of lymphatic and blood vessels.

The urinary system washes bacteria and other pathogens out of the bladder and urethra. The kidneys remove metabolic waste and other waste material resulting from phagocytosis in the bloodstream and secretes the waste into the bladder which excretes it in urine. The kidneys also help to maintain fluid balance in the body.

THE LYMPHATIC SYSTEM

Lymph

Lymph is a body fluid that consists of water, electrolytes, and proteins. Lymph also contains some of the other substances found in plasma, such as ions, nutrients, and gasses, but lymph contains more water than plasma. Lymph is initiated when blood pressure forces plasma out of the blood capillaries and into tissue spaces where it is called interstitial or intercellular fluid. Interstitial fluid bathes and nourishes the tissue cells and picks up microorganisms, foreign particles, enzymes, proteins, and hormones. Much of the interstitial fluid is reabsorbed into blood vessels, due to osmotic pressure, and the remaining interstitial fluid is absorbed from the tissue spaces into the initial lymphatics, where it is called lymph.

Lymph becomes more concentrated as it progresses through the lymphatic system, because water filters out through the vessels and nodes. Large molecules, like proteins and various cells, remain in the lymph vessels once they are absorbed from the tissues, and are carried through successively larger lymph vessels until they are delivered to the blood vessels in the **venous angle** at the clavicle.

Lymph Vessels

The lymph vessels, which include the initial lymphatics or lymph capillaries, the lymph vessels, **lymphatic trunks** and **lymphatic ducts**, form a network over the entire body to absorb fluid out of the tissues and through the lymph nodes. Lymph then travels through increasingly larger lymph vessels which finally connect with the cardiovascular system to channel the fluid into the bloodstream.

There are two levels of lymph circulation. Superficial vessels drain the skin and the mucosal tissues that are continuous with the skin and that line the digestive and respiratory tracts. Deeper vessels drain the muscles and internal organs. LDM directly affects the superficial circulation of lymph and indirectly affects the deep circulation of lymph because lymph flow is increased throughout the system as a result of massage. The lymphatic system begins in the tissues with the initial lymphatics, which are tiny one-way

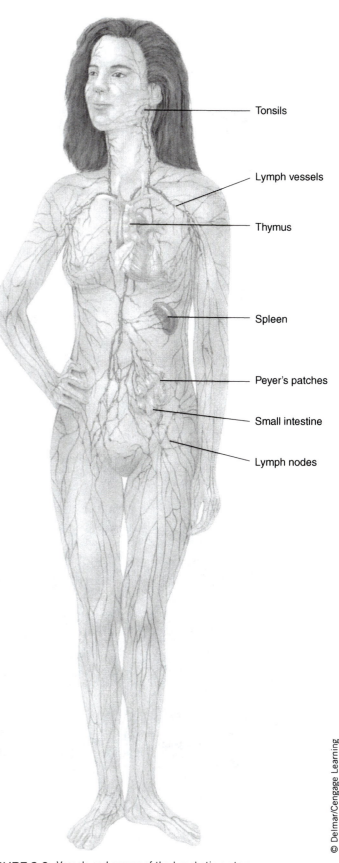

FIGURE 2-9 Vessels and organs of the lymphatic system

Tonsils
Lymph vessels
Thymus
Spleen
Peyer's patches
Small intestine
Lymph nodes

© Delmar/Cengage Learning

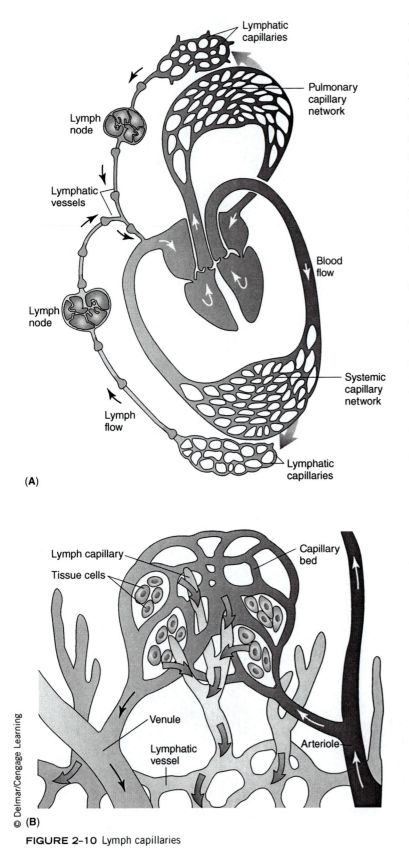

(A)

(B)

© Delmar/Cengage Learning

FIGURE 2–10 Lymph capillaries

vessels with closed ends (Figure 2–10). These vessels consist of a single layer of **endothelial cells** overlapping like thin leaflets. These overlapping cells form **flap valves**, little doorways that open to allow fluid to enter the lymphatic system. These cells are connected to the surrounding tissues by fibers. Body movement, including such gross anatomical movement as walking, heart beating, and intestinal peristalsis, causes these fibers to stretch and relax. As these fibers move, they pull the leaflike flaps open, allowing fluid to be absorbed into the lymphatic system.

Initial lymphatics differ from blood vessels. Blood capillaries are permeable, but the size of their openings is fixed and comparatively smaller than the openings of the initial lymphatics. This is because initial lymphatics lack the **basement membrane** that surrounds larger lymph vessels and blood vessels and gives them structure and strength (Figure 2–11). This makes initial lymphatics very loosely structured and very permeable. Openings to the initial lymphatics are variable and can widen when there is more fluid in the tissues.

Initial lymphatics also differ from blood vessels and larger lymph vessels in that initial lymphatics lack smooth muscle cells, and therefore, cannot contract.

From the initial lymphatics, lymph flows into larger lymph vessels called **precollectors**. Precollectors are larger than lymph capillaries, have some muscle cells in their walls, and are a little thicker. One to three layers of endothelial cells form the walls of the precollectors. Precollectors carry lymph away from tissues and toward lymph nodes. They are found in almost all tissues of the body, except the brain and spinal cord, bone marrow, and tissues without blood vessels, such as the epidermis and cartilage.

Like the valves in veins, precollecting vessels and lymph vessels are divided by bicuspid valves into segments called lymphangions. These valves prevent backward movement of the lymph when lymph vessels are compressed. These

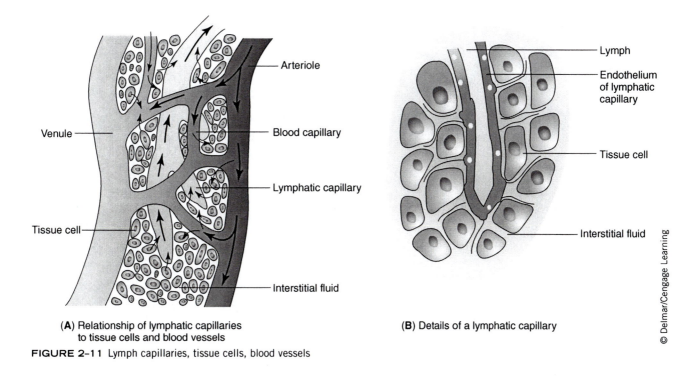

(A) Relationship of lymphatic capillaries
to tissue cells and blood vessels

(B) Details of a lymphatic capillary

FIGURE 2-11 Lymph capillaries, tissue cells, blood vessels

segments give the lymph vessels their characteristic beaded appearance. Each lymphangion can contract in response to an increase of tissue pressure inside it. As a lymphangion fills with fluid, it contracts, closing the flap valves through which fluid entered it and opening the flap valves leading to the next lymphangion. As the next lymphangion fills with fluid, it too contracts. This wavelike contraction of the lymphangions, similar to abdominal peristalsis, is the most important factor in the circulation of lymph.

Precollecting vessels and lymphatic vessels are most abundant near the inner and outer surfaces of the body, including the dermis (the outer skin layer) and the mucosal tissues (the inner surfaces lining the respiratory and digestive systems.) These areas are exposed to the environment around the body, and are more likely to contact disease-causing organisms. Lymph capillaries form a dense capillary bed very close to the surface of the skin. This is the layer that is most directly affected by LDM.

Precollecting vessels join to form larger lymph vessels or lymphatics, which resemble small veins. Lymph vessels carry lymph to the lymph nodes, and then to the **right lymphatic duct** and the thoracic duct. Like lymph capillaries, lymph vessels contain smooth muscle cells that contract in response to changes in fluid volume and pressure.

Lymph vessels that carry lymph toward the nodes are called **afferent vessels**; vessels that carry lymph out of the nodes and toward the lymphatic ducts are called **efferent vessels**. Each lymph node has more afferent vessels than efferent, which effectively slows lymph circulation at the nodes. Efferent vessels exit the lymph node at a depression on the side of the node called the hilum. Afferent vessels are attached at various areas on the surface of the lymph node.

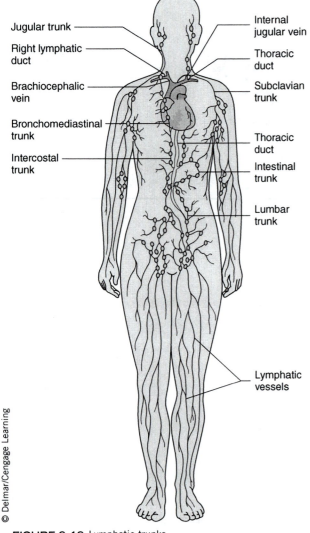

Jugular trunk

Right lymphatic duct

Brachiocephalic vein

Bronchomediastinal trunk

Intercostal trunk

Internal jugular vein

Thoracic duct

Subclavian trunk

Thoracic duct

Intestinal trunk

Lumbar trunk

Lymphatic vessels

FIGURE 2-12 Lymphatic trunks

After traveling through chains of lymph nodes, lymph is carried through larger and larger lymphatic vessels into lymphatic trunks. Lymphatic trunks drain large areas of the body and empty into the thoracic duct and the right lymphatic duct (Figure 2–12).

Lymphatic trunks carry lymph from large areas of the body to the lymphatic ducts. The **lumbar trunks** drain lymph from the legs, lower abdominal wall, and the pelvic organs; the **intestinal trunk** drains organs of the abdominal cavity; the intercostal and **bronchomediastinal trunks** receive lymph from portions of the thorax; the subclavian trunk drains the arm; and the **jugular trunk** drains parts of the neck and head. These trunks then join the thoracic duct or the right lymphatic duct.

The thoracic duct and the right lymphatic duct empty into jugular or subclavian veins in the venous angle above the clavicle. Lymph vessels from the right arm and the right half of the head, neck, and chest converge in the right lymphatic duct, which empties into the right subclavian vein. This structure does not exist in everyone; in many people, the large lymph vessels of the right upper quadrant merge and join blood vessels in the venous angle without forming a specific right lymphatic duct.

Lymph vessels from the left arm and the left side of the head, neck, and chest empty into the thoracic duct. The thoracic duct is located in the thoracic cavity and arises from the cisterna chyli, a collecting vessel that receives lymph from the abdomen and fluid from the small intestines, an emulsion of lymph and fat molecules called **chyle** that is formed during digestion. The thoracic duct empties into the left venous angle, connecting to the subclavian or jugular vein. Lymph vessels from both lower limbs and the abdominal cavity also empty into the thoracic duct after passing through the lymph nodes (Figure 2–13).

Lymph Nodes

Lymph nodes are specialized collections of lymph tissue located along the lymphatic vessels (Figure 2–8). Superficial nodes are mainly concentrated in the inguinal, cervical, and axillary regions. There are smaller groups near the elbows and knees. Deep nodes are located far down into the abdomen, near the lumbar vertebrae, and connected to the small intestines. Some deep nodes are found in the liver.

Lymph nodes are covered by fibrous connective tissue that extends into the node, dividing it into compartments called sinuses. The outer portion of each compartment is called the cortex of the node. The cortex contains dense clusters of lymphocytes called lymph nodules. The center of each cluster is called the germinal center, which is where lymphocytes reproduce by cell division. The inner part of a lymph node is called the medulla. Strands of lymphocytes from the cortex extend into the medulla.

White blood cells are trapped inside lymph nodes. As lymph filters through lymph nodes, white blood cells identify and destroy microorganisms and microscopic foreign particles that may harm the body. As it comes from the cell spaces into the initial lymphatics, lymph is contaminated. After it has passed through the lymph nodes to be returned to the blood circulatory system, lymph is sterile.

When white blood cells identify **antigens**, the white blood cells multiply rapidly, causing the lymph node to swell (Figure 2–14). The enlarged lymph node may be painful, but it is a sign that the immune system is doing its job. Lymph nodes have more efferent vessels (the vessels leading into the node) than afferent vessels (the vessels that exit the node.) This causes lymph circulation to slow down, allowing the **phagocytes** in the lymph node time to recognize and attack pathogens.

In the presence of inflammation or infection, lymph nodes can be swollen, painful and usually moveable. After the infection or inflammation is resolved, the lymph node returns to its normal size, unless there is scar tissue in the node itself, in which case the lymph node may remain enlarged. If a tumor develops in the lymph node, it becomes enlarged but may not be painful. It may also become fixed (can't be moved with palpation) due to the tumor connecting to the surrounding tissues. It is impossible to know what an enlarged lymph node means by palpation alone. Therapists and estheticians should always recommend that their clients with enlarged nodes have them examined by a doctor.

Normally, it is difficult to palpate lymph nodes, as they are small, soft and not tender, except in the presence of infection, inflammation or tumor growth. In order to locate lymph nodes, knowledge of lymph anatomy is important. Using knowledge of lymph anatomy, the therapist or esthetician palpates in the areas where lymph nodes can be found. Lymph nodes can't always be found by palpation, which is normal. If lymph nodes can be felt, they may be full of white blood cells responding to attack, or they may be scarred due to previous infection and inflammation. They may also be enlarged due to tumor

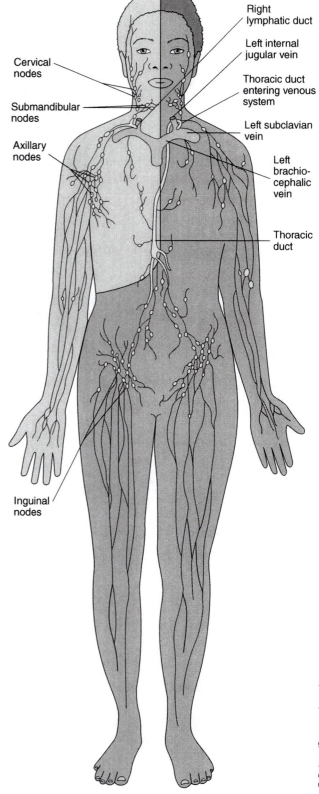

FIGURE 2-13 Ducts

Cervical nodes
Submandibular nodes
Axillary nodes
Inguinal nodes

Right lymphatic duct
Left internal jugular vein
Thoracic duct entering venous system
Left subclavian vein
Left brachio-cephalic vein
Thoracic duct

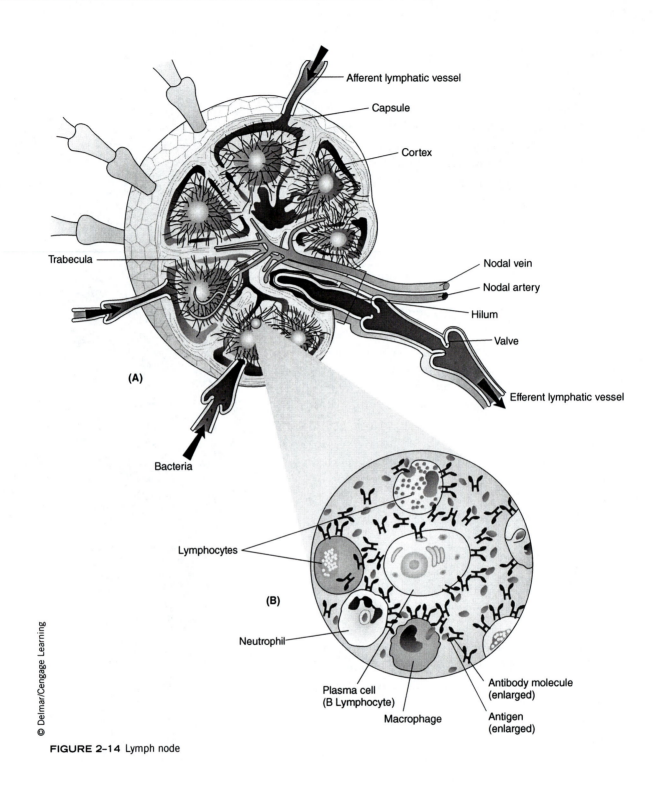

Afferent lymphatic vessel

Capsule

Cortex

Nodal vein

Nodal artery

Hilum

Valve

Trabecula

(A)

Efferent lymphatic vessel

Bacteria

Lymphocytes

(B)

Neutrophil

Antibody molecule
(enlarged)

Plasma cell
(B Lymphocyte)

Antigen
(enlarged)

Macrophage

FIGURE 2-14 Lymph node

growth. If nodes can be identified by palpation, ask the client whether he or she has ever had them examined by a doctor. If not, then recommend that the client do so on their next visit to a physician.

LYMPH ORGANS

Lymph organs include the **tonsils**, thymus, spleen, and **Peyer's patches**. Lymph nodes, lymph nodules (Peyer's patches), and tonsils are collections of lymph tissue that filter lymph, destroying microorganisms that may be dangerous to the body. Lymph nodules are found in the respiratory and digestive tracts, areas where there is more potential exposure to disease-causing agents. Tonsils are located in a ring around the openings to the respiratory and digestive tracts. There are collections of lymph nodes in the neck, **axilla**, and groin. The spleen, a large lymph node located along blood vessels rather than lymph vessels, is considered the lymph node of the blood. Immune reactions can occur anywhere in the body, but the lymph nodes and the spleen are where most action takes place.

Tonsils

The tonsils form a ring of **lymphatic tissue** that surrounds the opening to the digestive and respiratory tracts, an area where harmful substances can easily enter the body (Figure 2–6). Tonsils are lymph nodes, but they lack afferent vessels. Instead of having lymph fluid delivered to them via the lymph vessels, tonsils have compartments containing lymphoid tissue that can sense foreign bacteria that enter the body through the mouth and nose, and destroy them.

There are three pairs of tonsils: (1) pharyngeal, (2) palatine, and (3) lingual. The palatine tonsils are often removed surgically (via tonsillectomy) when they are chronically infected. Pharyngeal tonsils, often called **adenoids**, are also occasionally removed when they become infected and obstruct breathing. Lingual tonsils are rarely removed. The lymphatic system can withstand removal of the tonsils, because although the tonsils are the first line of defense for the openings of the respiratory and digestive tracts, those tracts are also lined with nodules of lymph tissue and a rich bed of lymph capillaries and vessels that contain lymphocytes to fight disease.

Spleen

The spleen, the largest organ of the lymphatic system, acts as the lymph node of the blood. Like other lymph nodes, the spleen traps and manufactures lymphocytes. Instead of filtering lymph, the spleen filters blood. The spleen contains white and red pulp. Blood is filtered through the red pulp, where dying red blood cells are phagocytized, or broken down into parts, some of which the body reuses. **Macrophages** in the white pulp destroy dangerous microorganisms and foreign substances.

Thymus

The thymus is a two-lobed organ located in the thorax over the heart. It is similar in construction to a lymph node, with a cortex and a medulla. An endocrine gland, the thymus helps newborns and young children develop **antibodies** and decreases in size with age. It shrinks after puberty, but continues to be an active part of the immune system. Immature lymphocytes that are produced in the red bone marrow migrate to the thymus, where they develop into **T-cells**. The thymus produces a group of hormones called thymosins, which have extremely varied biological functions. It is believed that thymosins help T-cells mature. T-cells circulate in the bloodstream and are transported to the lymph nodes via blood vessels connected with the nodes.

Aggregated lymph nodules are collections of lymph tissue in the mucus tissues lining the respiratory and digestive tracts. These areas include the tonsils, the bronchi of the respiratory tract, the small intestine, and the appendix. Lymphocytes in aggregated lymph nodules respond to antigens (a toxin or foreign microorganism that produces an immune response) in those areas and create antibodies. The openings to the respiratory and digestive tracts, the nose and mouth, allow antigens to easily enter the body. Aggregated lymph nodules are located to help rapidly overcome the antigens as soon as they enter the body.

REVIEW QUESTIONS

1. Describe lymph. What is its source, and how does it differ from interstitial fluid?
2. How do initial lymphatics differ from lymph vessels?
3. What are lymphatic ducts? How many are there?
4. Describe a lymph node. How does it help protect against disease?
5. In which two ways do lymph capillaries differ from blood capillaries?
6. Into which large veins do the lymphatic ducts empty?
7. What is the function of the bicuspid valves in the lymph vessels?
8. The thoracic duct receives lymph fluid from which areas of the body?
9. What is the difference between afferent and efferent lymph vessels?
10. Where are the tonsils located, and how many are there?
11. What is the function of the tonsils?
12. How do tonsils differ from other lymph nodes?
13. Which lymphatic organ stores blood? What are its other functions?
14. Where is the thymus located?
15. What role does the thymus play in the lymphatic system?
16. Describe the location of lymph nodules and the purpose they serve.
17. How do initial lymphatic vessels differ from lymph capillaries?

Lymph Circulation

L ymph circulation differs from blood circulation because the lymphatic system lacks a central pump like the heart. Lymph circulation depends on other factors, including muscle contraction, skeletal movement, internal and external changes in pressure, spontaneous contractility of lymph vessels, and external factors such as massage and gravity. The most important factor in lymph circulation is the **lymphatic pump**, the rhythmic, wavelike contractions of the lymphangions.

Lymph circulation involves two distinct steps or stages:

1. lymph absorption into the initial lymphatics and capillaries
2. propulsion of lymph through the network of contractile lymphatic vessels

INITIAL LYMPHATICS

The lymphatic system drains all regions of the body. Lymph drainage begins with channels between cells in our skin, muscles, and other tissues. Tissue fluid finds its way to the initial lymphatics in the same way that a flash flood in the desert creates channels in the sand, small channels that move water toward larger channels, streams, and even rivers.

The channels between tissue cells drain toward initial lymphatics, very tiny vessels with ends that open into tissue spaces. Although initial lymphatics look like blood vessels, there are striking differences. Blood vessels have a well-defined basement membrane, an outer wall of connective tissue that gives them structure and resilience. These blood vessel membranes are fenestrated, or honeycombed with windows, through which plasma, proteins, and red blood cells escape from the blood to the cell spaces in tissues and organs.

Initial lymphatics, in contrast, are structured more loosely. Because of this, proteins and other components of tissue fluid can enter the lymphatic system easily. They enter through gaps between endothelial cells in the initial lymphatics. The endothelial cells of the initial lymphatics resemble leaves and are connected to surrounding structures by microfilaments. As tissue fluid pressure increases, the gaps between the endothelial cells widen. This allows tissue fluid, with its components, to enter the lymphatics.[1] Body movements like walking, yawning, and stretching, which cause the skin to move, trigger the stretch reflex of the initial lymphatics.

Initial lymphatics are completely enmeshed in and are part of the connective tissue layer immediately below the skin, which also contains fat cells, blood vessels, and nerve cells. The microfilaments that connect the initial lymphatics to surrounding tissues stretch and relax as the skin moves. As the microfilaments stretch and relax, they tug on the endothelial cells in the initial lymphatics, pulling them open and allowing tissue fluid to flow in.

OTHER FACTORS THAT DRIVE LYMPH CIRCULATION

Other factors that affect lymph drainage include voluntary body movements, walking, stretching, and dancing. Involuntary body movements such as abdominal peristalsis, respiration, arterial pulse, and contractions of local muscles all stimulate lymph circulation. These factors cause the overlapping cells of the initial lymphatics to pull open, and stimulate the lymph vessels to contract.[2,3,4]

Lymph circulation is also affected by local fluid dynamics. As the volume of fluid in the tissues increases, it fills the spaces between the tissue cells and moves them farther apart. Also, as the volume of fluid in the tissues increases, pressure increases. Fluid tends to move from areas with more pressure to areas with less pressure, in an attempt at equalization. Blood pressure forces fluid out of blood vessels, increasing tissue pressure. As tissue pressure increases, the endothelial cells that cover the openings to the initial lymphatics move apart and fluid can enter the lymphatic system, increasing fluid pressure and volume inside them.[5,6]

The Lymphatic Pump

From the initial lymphatics, lymph moves into larger lymph capillaries, divided into sections called lymphangions. Increased pressure inside the lymphangions causes them to contract, propelling lymph forward through larger and larger lymphatic vessels, and eventually into the nearest lymph nodes.[7,8] These wave-like contractions continue beyond the lymph nodes, as lymph fluid continues to drain into larger and larger vessels, eventually draining toward the lymphatic ducts.

Contractions of the lymphatics are not coordinated with the heart or breath rate,[9] but are related to factors in the lymphatic system. Lymphatic contractions start and stop depending on whether the pressure inside the lymphangions exceeds or falls below certain levels. When pressure in the tissues becomes too great, lymph circulation in the area stops and edema develops. Edema is a sign that lymph circulation has decreased or stopped in the area.

Exercise

During exercise, lymphatic circulation inside muscles increases up to 15 times the resting rate. Exercise has the effect of scrubbing the muscles clean. At first, the lymphatic fluid from the muscles is full of proteins, dead red blood cells, and waste material from the muscle cells. As exercise continues, the muscles continue to alternately contract and relax, propelling lymph through the vessels and pulling fluid from the muscle tissues. Gradually, the lymph contains fewer and fewer such particles.[10] The fluid that is removed from the muscles via the lymphatic system is replaced with more fluid from local blood vessels, containing nutrients for muscle cells. However, vigorous exercise that stimulates lymph circulation in muscles is only a small part of the entire lymph circulation of the body. Many lymph vessels are located in the skin and in tissues contiguous with the skin, such as the digestive and respiratory tracts, and the contraction of voluntary skeletal muscles does not affect these superficial vessels directly.

Breathing

During inhalation, the thoracic duct is squeezed, pushing fluid forward, toward the venous angle, and creating a partial vacuum in the duct. During exhalation, fluid is pulled from lymphatic vessels into the thoracic duct to fill the vacuum created by inhalation. Other natural movements inside the body, such as abdominal peristalsis and the beating of the heart, affect lymph vessels and stimulate lymph movement. Pressure inside the chest cavity is less than atmospheric pressure outside the body. This creates a slight vacuum in the chest cavity that helps draw lymph into the thoracic duct.[11,12,13]

Gentle Body Movements

Low-amplitude body movements, such as walking 40 paces per minute, and such natural movements as blinking, yawning, sneezing, and stretching, help to empty lymphatics in the chest and abdomen, which then draw in fluid from the lymphatics in the periphery.[14] Inactivity can contribute to lymph stasis (edema). Then, tissue fluid tends to pool in lower regions of the body in response to gravity. One example is the painful swollen legs experienced by many who take long international flights during which they must sit in one place for hours at a time. Lymph circulation slows during rest. Stretching and yawning upon awakening stimulate lymph circulation.

Variations in Pressure

Plasma is forced out of blood capillaries because the blood pressure there is greater than the pressure in the surrounding tissues. Increased fluid volume in the cellular spaces of surrounding tissues (interstitia) causes cells to move apart, straining the microscopic fibers that connect the endothelial cells of the initial lymphatics to tissue cells. The pull on the microfilaments causes the endothelial cells to open like flaps, allowing tissue fluid to enter the initial lymphatics. The pressure of the accumulating fluid in the initial lymphatics forces lymph through one-way valves and into larger lymph capillaries.

External Mechanical Factors

Massage and passive movement increase lymph flow and the rate of contractions of the lymphatic vessels.[15] Massage mechanically moves fluid, like squeezing water through a tube. It also stimulates the lymph vessels to contract, starting the lymphatic pump so that lymph circulation will continue on its own.

Passive movement, when the therapist helps the client move the arms and legs, also helps to stimulate lymph circulation, a real benefit to those immobilized by injury and paralysis. Similarly, limb elevation allows gravity to function so that lymph flows away from the limb.[16,17] To be most effective, the arms and legs must be properly elevated. If the knees are elevated but the ankles and feet are not, lymph from the lower leg will not drain as effectively. With the client lying in a supine position, the ankles must be propped up slightly higher than the knees, which must be a little higher than the hip joint. The hip joint should be only slightly flexed to prevent compressing lymphatics in the region of the joint. Similarly, when elevating the arm, the hand must be slightly higher than the elbow, which in turn must be slightly higher than the shoulder.

LYMPH DRAINAGE PATHWAYS

Lymph circulation begins in the periphery, in the tissues just below the skin. The body is divided into **lymphotomes**, four quarters of the trunk, each with an attached limb. They are the right and left upper quadrants, and the right and left lower quadrants. The lymphotomes are divided vertically at the midline, and horizontally at the level of the navel and the 5th lumbar vertebra. The anastomoses at the margins of each quadrant are often called **watersheds**. At the margins of each quadrant, lymphatics overlap with drainage across the watersheds. As a result, tissue fluid can be drained from a congested area to an adjacent quadrant where it can enter the lymphatic system.

Therapists can take advantage of the watersheds, noting not only changes in the tissue in the area being massaged, but also noting the direction in which the fluid moves, following the movement of the fluid around obstructions toward lymph nodes. This of course takes practice and well-developed palpation skills.

REVIEW QUESTIONS

1. List at least three factors that affect lymph circulation.
2. What are the two stages of lymph circulation?
3. Describe differences between the structure of lymph and blood vessels.
4. What is the lymphatic pump?
5. Describe the effects of exercise on lymph circulation.
6. Which factors can hinder lymph circulation?
7. The lymphatic system is part of what larger system?

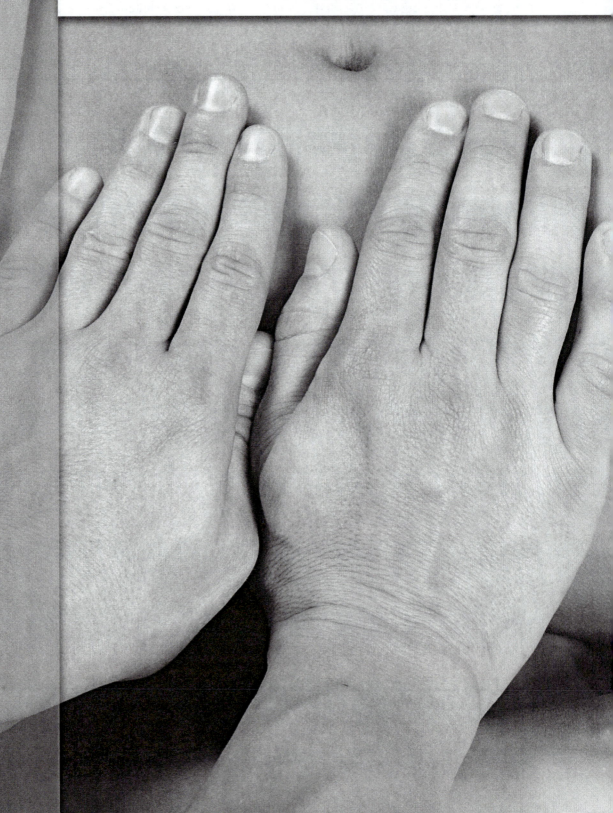

Functions of the Lymphatic System

The lymphatic system has a number of important functions.[1] It removes fluid from tissues and returns it to the blood circulatory system. The lymphatic system distributes immune cells throughout the body to maintain health and defend against disease. The lymphatic system also rids tissues of excess proteins and toxins, and carries digested fat from the intestines to the blood vessels. It helps to repair damage in injured tissues. The lymphatic system can also regenerate and even develop new lymph nodes in areas of chronic infection.

IMMUNITY

The lymphatic system is the first line of defense against disease on a cellular level. The lymphatic system helps to transport immune cells throughout the body. Also, lymph nodes filter lymph and the spleen filters blood. These organs contain lymphocytes that can recognize and destroy microorganisms which threaten the organism. The success of the lymphatic system depends on the ability of the immune cells to differentiate between cells that belong to the body and invaders that do not. It also depends on the ability of immune cells to create antibodies. Immune cells create antibodies for each disease organism they encounter. For the rest of a person's life, the immune system will recognize and destroy those organisms each time they invade.

MAINTAIN BLOOD PRESSURE, BLOOD VOLUME, AND FLUID BALANCE

The lymphatic system helps to maintain a healthy balance of fluid volume and pressure in both the tissues and the cardiovascular system. Under normal circumstances, fluid is removed from tissues and returned to blood vessels continuously, helping to maintain tissue fluid volume, blood volume, and blood pressure. A large volume of fluid washes in and out of blood into the body's tissues every day. That fluid, which is basically plasma and contains proteins, lymph cells, red blood cells, electrolytes, and nutrients, washes the spaces between tissue cells. It also is absorbed into cells, picking up microorganisms, microscopic particles, and metabolic waste from cells. About 90 percent of that fluid is absorbed back into the bloodstream through blood capillaries, which are permeable. The remaining 10 percent, about three liters,[2] enters the **lymphatic capillaries** and passes through the lymphatic system before returning to the blood via the subclavian veins.

PREVENTING PROTEIN BUILDUP IN TISSUES

Although most of the fluid that filters out of blood vessels into tissues is reabsorbed into the bloodstream, large molecules and cells are not reabsorbed. The openings in blood capillaries are relatively small compared to the openings in the initial lymphatics. The lymphatic system has the capability to absorb these large molecules and cells, removing them from tissues and returning them to the cardiovascular system. Left in the tissues, proteins can trigger an inflammatory response and the side effects of pain, swelling and scar tissue formation. Eventually, protein buildup in tissues can be life threatening, so this function of the lymphatic system is vital. The lymphatic system also absorbs foreign microorganisms and particles from tissues and passes all these substances through the lymph nodes, where they are destroyed before the lymph returns to the bloodstream.

DISTRIBUTING DIETARY FAT

The lymphatic system transports fats from the small intestines to the bloodstream through the lymphatics and the thoracic duct. Special lymph vessels called **lacteals** are located in the lining of the small intestine. **Chyle** is a milky fluid consisting of emulsified fat droplets and lymph that is extracted from chyme, a mixture of gastric juices and partially digested food. During digestion, the chyle drains from the lacteals and passes through the lymph vessels into the veins near the heart.

HEALING INJURIES

The lymphatic system also helps to repair the damage from injured tissues. When there is an injury to tissue, such as the skin or a muscle, chemicals from the damaged cells cause inflammation. Blood circulation in the area increases, and capillaries become more permeable. More fluid is released into the damaged area, bringing with it immune cells and fibers that start to wall off the area and destroy any dangerous microorganisms. The pressure difference between the fluid-filled tissues and the lymphatic vessels creates a slight vacuum that pulls debris from the injury, including dead cells, microorganisms, and foreign particles, into the initial lymphatics and eventually to the lymph nodes, where it is destroyed.

NEW AREAS OF RESEARCH

One of the amazing abilities of the lymphatic system, only recently recognized and not yet studied in depth, is its powers of regeneration. The sprouting of new lymph capillaries in areas where lymph flow has been disrupted has been observed, as well as the growth of new lymph nodes in areas of chronic infection. It appears that new lymph nodes can grow along deep lymph vessels in the extremities when normal lymph nodes are scarred and damaged by chronic infection.[3]

In spite of the difficulty of studying the lymphatic system in living persons, recent developments such as magnetic resonance imaging (MRI) and microsurgical techniques, as well as the demand from lymphedema patients for more research, have contributed to knowledge of the lymphatic system and will aid continued research.[4]

REVIEW QUESTIONS

1. What are the main functions of the lymphatic system?
2. Why is it important that proteins are removed from tissues, and why are the blood vessels unable to absorb proteins from tissues?
3. How does dietary fat enter the bloodstream and pass through the heart?
4. What role does the lymphatic system play when there is an injury to a tissue like the skin or muscles?
5. What role does the lymphatic system play when someone is exposed to a disease-causing microorganism?
6. How does the lymphatic system affect blood volume?
7. What is the most important function of the lymphatic system?

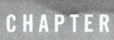

CHAPTER 5

Immunity

I mmunity is the body's ability to resist damage from microorganisms and other foreign substances, like harmful chemicals. The human body has **nonspecific** and **specific** systems to defend against microorganisms and harmful substances. Nonspecific immunity is innate, but specific immunity, which must be **acquired**, depends on the ability of immune cells to produce antibodies.

NONSPECIFIC IMMUNITY

Nonspecific immunity or "innate resistance" includes mechanical methods of resistance, chemicals, the inflammatory response, and macrophages, all of which provide barriers to foreign substances. Humans are born with nonspecific mechanisms to defend against disease.

Mechanical Methods of Resistance

Mechanical processes prevent microorganisms from entering the body, or they remove microorganisms from the body. For example, the cells of the dermis and epidermis create a barrier that prevents microorganisms from entering the body. The acidity and high fat content of skin contribute to this process by inhibiting the growth of microorganisms. Another example is the sticky mucus produced by the mucous membranes. This mucus traps microorganisms and moves them out of the body. Tears, saliva, and urine wash away microorganisms, while nasal hairs filter air during inhalation. The cilia of the upper respiratory tract sweep microorganisms up so that they are coughed up and can be swallowed. Then they enter the digestive tract, where they are destroyed by acid in the stomach. All these entities, without differentiating between bacteria, viruses or molds, react to invaders in the same way.

Chemical Resistance

Chemical resistance includes nonspecific antiviral and antibacterial substances produced by the body. Some chemicals on the surfaces of cells destroy microorganisms or prevent their entry into cells. Lysozyme in tears and saliva, sebum on skin, and mucus on the mucous membranes are such chemicals. Interferon protects cells against viral infections by preventing viral replication.

INFLAMMATION

The inflammatory response (Figure 5–1) occurs when injuries, infections, poisons, and the like damage tissues. Inflammation is characterized by redness, heat, swelling, and pain. Increased blood flow to the injured area causes the typical symptoms of redness and heat. Chemicals released by injured cells cause vasodilation and increased permeability of local blood vessels. As a result, more fluid is extravasated into the injured tissues. The pressure of the fluid on nerve receptors causes swelling (edema) and pain. The chemical signals released by injured cells also attract leukocytes, which can move toward the site of tissue damage, in a process called chemotaxis. There, the leukocytes begin to destroy invading cells, foreign particles, and dead or damaged cells.

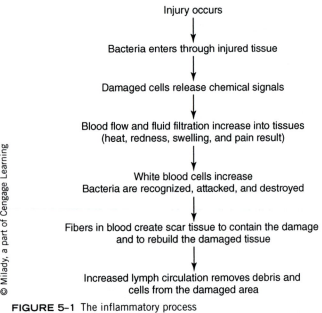

Injury occurs

↓

Bacteria enters through injured tissue

↓

Damaged cells release chemical signals

↓

Blood flow and fluid filtration increase into tissues
(heat, redness, swelling, and pain result)

↓

White blood cells increase
Bacteria are recognized, attacked, and destroyed

↓

Fibers in blood create scar tissue to contain the damage
and to rebuild the damaged tissue

↓

Increased lymph circulation removes debris and
cells from the damaged area

FIGURE 5–1 The inflammatory process

© Milady, a part of Cengage Learning

The first cells to reach a damaged area are **neutrophils**, which immediately begin destroying invading cells. These are followed by macrophages. Macrophages are **monocytes** that escape the bloodstream into the tissues and grow. They are phagocytes, which means they destroy invading cells by surrounding and covering them, absorbing them and then breaking them into particles. Phagocytosis is the process by which phagocytes digest and break down foreign cells.

Along with the immune cells, fibroblasts migrate to the area of injury and begin to build scar tissue to isolate the injured tissue from healthy tissue, and to rebuild the damaged tissue.

Lymphatic circulation increases as local lymphatic capillaries begin absorbing tissue fluid, red blood cells (erythrocytes), and proteins spilled from damaged blood vessels. The local lymphatics absorb interstitial fluid, as well as dead or damaged cells, invading cells, and foreign particles, bringing them into contact with more immune cells in the lymph nodes.

One of the effects of inflammation is "splinting," as the swelling caused by the injury helps to immobilize the injured area, protecting against further injury. Therapists should recognize that swelling following an injury or strain may be concealing a more serious problem such as a fracture or tear. Delay lymph drainage massage until after the client has been examined by a physician to rule out internal injuries.

SPECIFIC IMMUNITY

While nonspecific defenses of the body resist against all attackers in the same way, specific immunity defenses of the immune system will recognize and destroy specific foreign microorganisms. Specific immunity depends on exposure to antigens and disease-causing cells, and on antibody production. In a lifetime, the body's approximately 2 trillion lymphocytes can produce 100 million trillion antibodies, each targeted at a different invading microorganism. Antibodies are developed after the body is exposed to a foreign substance for the first time. They remain in the system for decades, and can remember the foreign substance and attack it more quickly after the next exposure. One example of this activity is the immunity that results from certain childhood diseases, like mumps, measles, and chicken pox.

A very important factor in specific immunity is the body's ability to recognize the difference between self-cells and not-self cells, and to destroy only the not-self cells (invading microbes that cause disease). **Autoimmune diseases** occur when the body becomes confused, and the immune system starts to attack self-cells as if they were foreign invaders.

ACQUIRED IMMUNITY

Antibody-based immunity is acquired as the organism is exposed to a multitude of attacking foreign microorganisms over a lifetime.

1. **Active immunity** or natural acquired immunity results from everyday exposure to antigens against which the body's immune system responds. As humans age, they develop more and more antibodies to different kinds of microorganisms, develop better resistance, and therefore fall ill less often than children.
2. Active artificial immunity results from deliberate exposure to an antigen by means of a vaccine. Weak or dead disease-causing microorganisms are injected, and the body develops antibodies that recognize these microorganisms quickly when again exposed to them.
3. **Passive immunity** or natural immunity refers to the transfer of antibodies from a mother to her fetus or baby through the umbilical cord during gestation and through nursing. This helps to protect infants and children until they develop their own antibodies.
4. Passive artificial immunity is the transfer of antibodies from an animal or another person to a person requiring immunity. This medical procedure helps those with impaired immune systems who are producing too few antibodies. For example, in the case of rabies or tetanus exposure, the immune system is not able to overcome the disease pathogen quickly enough for survival, so an injection of antibodies against these diseases from another person provides immediate protection and allows the immune system time to develop its own antibodies.

CATEGORIZING CELLS

The purpose of the lymphatic system is to protect the body against the harmful effects of invading microorganisms, poisons, and dead or dying cells. The lymphatic system has its own cells for this purpose. It consists of stationary cells, which make up the tissue of the lymph organs, and moving cells, which migrate throughout the body by means of body fluids: plasma, interstitial fluid, and lymph. As a group, the moving cells are called white blood cells, or leukocytes.

White blood cells, or leukocytes, are formed in red bone marrow, and reproduce in blood and lymph tissue. After leaving the bone marrow through the blood vessels, these cells enter tissues and eventually filter into the lymphatic system. There are six types of leukocytes, each with specific functions. Scientists have classified white blood cells into two groups–granulocytes and agranulocytes–depending on whether or not granules are seen when the cells are stained with a dye and viewed under a light microscope. There are three types of granulocytes, which contain the granules: neutrophils, eosinophils and basophils. There are three types of agranulocytes, which lack granules in their cellular cytoplasm: lymphocytes, monocytes, and macrophages. Under the category of lymphocytes are the B-cells, T-cells and NK cells.

Neutrophils

Neutrophils are usually the first cells to reach damaged areas, moving by chemotaxis and attracted due to the chemical signal emitted by damaged cells. Neutrophils ingest bacteria and other substances through phagocytosis. After ingesting only a few microorganisms, neutrophils die readily, creating pus. Pus is a thick, opaque liquid composed of dead neutrophils. Neutrophils compose about 60 to 70 percent of the leukocytes in the body.

Monocytes and Macrophages

Monocytes are immature macrophages that travel in blood and lymph. They can pass through the walls of the blood and lymphatic system and mature into macrophages, about five times larger than monocytes. Macrophages, phagocytes that travel to damaged tissue after neutrophils, are responsible for most of the activity in the later stages of infection. Macrophages clean up dead neutrophils and other cellular debris, as well as destroy microorganisms and foreign substances. They destroy many more cells before dying than do neutrophils, and they are also found in uninfected tissues such as the skin, mucous membranes, blood and lymphatic vessels, lymph nodes, and the spleen, where they phagocytize microorganisms before they can cause damage or reproduce. Macrophages do not produce antibodies, but are part of the nonspecific immune system.

Basophils

Basophils release histamine, leukotrienes and prostaglandins in order to trigger inflammation, increase capillary permeability and increase mucus production in response to the presence of microbes. Basophils account for about 1 percent of leukocytes. Mast cells are cells that are filled with basophil granules, and they also release histamine during inflammatory and allergic reactions.

Eosinophils

Eosinophils release chemicals that reduce inflammation. Eosinophils account for about 1 to 4 percent of leukocytes.

Natural Killer Cells

Natural killer (NK) cells are a type of leukocyte produced in red bone marrow, composing about 1 to 3 percent of all lymphocytes. NK cells do not exhibit specificity or memory but recognize and destroy a general class of cells, such as tumor cells.

B- and T-lymphocytes

B- and T-lymphocytes produce antibodies and other, similar chemicals responsible for destroying microorganisms, particularly viruses (Figure 5–2).

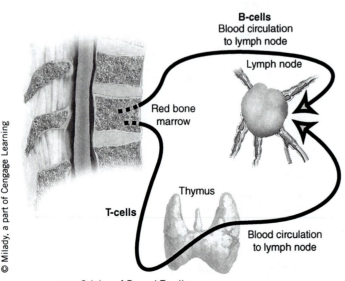

B-cells
Blood circulation
to lymph node

Lymph node

Red bone
marrow

Thymus

T-cells

Blood circulation
to lymph node

FIGURE 5-2 Origins of B- and T-cells

Lymphocytes contribute to allergic reactions, graft and transplant rejections, tumor control, and immune system regulation. Lymphocytes account for 20 to 30 percent of leukocytes.

B- and T-lymphocytes originate in red bone marrow. **B-cells** mature in bone marrow, but T-cells travel to the thymus first. The thymus secretes hormones that mature the cells into T-cells before they are distributed throughout the body. There are about five T-cells for every B-cell, and both cells circulate constantly through the blood and lymph, although they remain most of the time in the lymph organs. B-cells produce antibodies and protect against bacteria, toxins, and viruses outside of cells. T-cells help B-cells, and kill cells containing viruses and tumor cells.

REVIEW QUESTIONS

1. How does nonspecific immunity differ from specific immunity?
2. Specific immunity depends on what two factors?
3. What is an antibody?
4. What is an antigen?
5. How does inflammation protect the body from disease?
6. In what four ways can specific immunity be acquired?
7. Give two examples of nonspecific immunity.
8. Describe three lymphocytes.
9. Is there a difference between a monocyte and a macrophage?
10. Give an example of mechanical resistance to disease.
11. Give an example of chemical resistance.

6

Edema

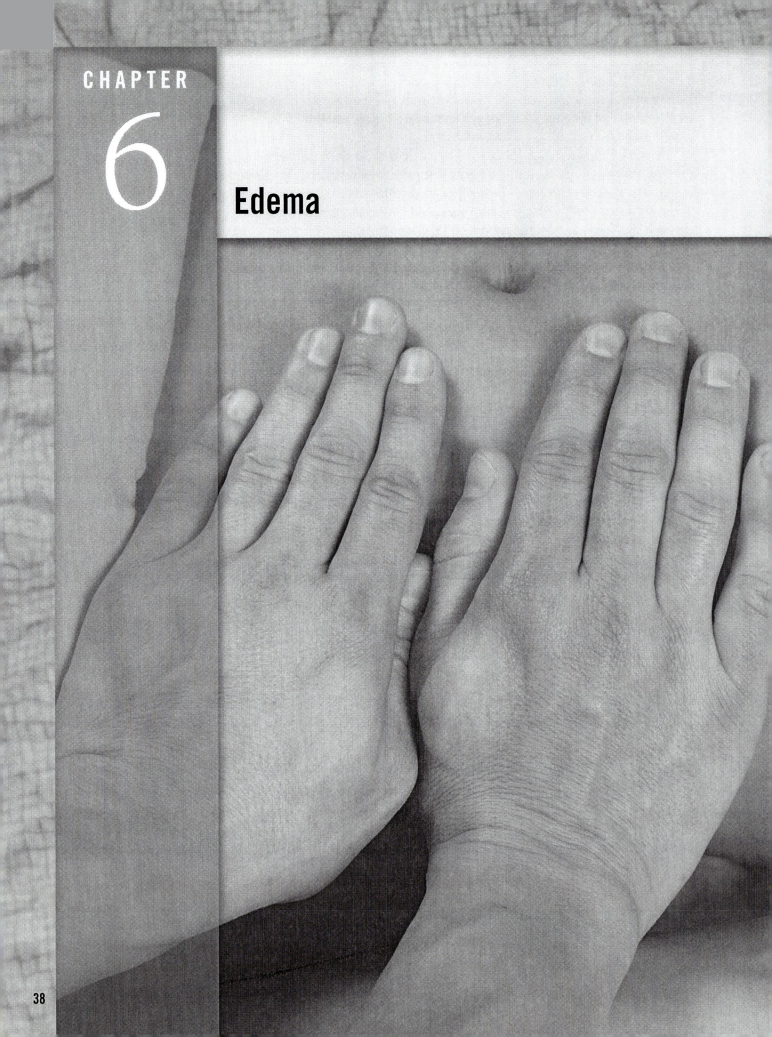

Edema is a condition in which excess interstitial fluid saturates tissues, causing swelling. Edema is generally a temporary condition. Chronic edema is called lymphedema disease. Edema means that lymphatic flow in that area is overloaded.[1] When lymphatic function is overloaded, it is either because the load is too great (the amount of fluid in the tissues exceeds the capacity of the lymphatics), or function has been lost (e.g., lymph vessels are damaged or missing, lymph nodes may have been removed, or scar tissue may be blocking lymph circulation). Edema and lymphedema are usually due to obstruction in the lymph vessels or lymph nodes. Obstruction can be due to injury, surgery, removal of lymph nodes, radiation therapy, or infections. Obstruction can also be due to a tumor of the lymphatics or the lymph nodes.

Lymph obstruction prevents drainage of tissue fluid into the lymphatic system, so the fluid accumulates in subcutaneous tissue, between fat cells and the connective tissue fibers holding the fat cells in place, as well as inside and outside muscular fascia. As the amount of fluid increases in subcutaneous tissue, it forms interconnecting channels between the fat cells, as a flash flood creates flood channels in desert sand.[2,3]

UNDERSTANDING EDEMA BASICS

Edema can be a simple and temporary problem due to various factors, such as too much salt in the diet, which causes fluid retention. A sedentary lifestyle can lead to edema, because there is too little activity to stimulate lymph circulation. Lymph circulation is stimulated by muscle contraction and relaxation, and by low-amplitude body movements. When the body is still and there is little activity, lymph circulation decreases and fluid that would normally absorb into the lymphatic system instead pools in the interstitia or tissue spaces. Tissue fluids also respond to gravity, so inactivity can cause these fluids to pool in the legs, ankles, and lower areas of the body.

As part of the inflammatory response, edema can also result from such minor injuries as contusions or burns. Injured tissue cells send chemical signals that increase the local blood flow and make the blood vessels more permeable. As a result, more fluid filters out into the damaged area, causing swelling. Local lymphatic vessels may be damaged, decreasing their capacity to remove fluid from the area. Scar tissue that develops after an injury can block lymphatic circulation, causing edema. In fact, experienced massage therapists often observe small edematous areas on their clients' bodies that coexist with scar tissue and damage from previous injuries. For instance, many people who have sprained their ankles, even years before, will have chronic swelling around the injured ankles.

Edema may also occur over tissues that are stiff due to emotional trauma. Stress and the fight-or-flight physiologic response cause muscles to tighten and to remain tight. Massage therapists, estheticians, and others who perform LDM often observe this combination of tissue conditions: chronic muscle stiffness and lymph stasis due to stress.

Lack of Exercise

Exercise in which muscles alternately contract and relax will stimulate lymph circulation in the muscle and cleanse muscle tissue. Muscle contraction and relaxation will also affect nearby lymph vessels, stimulating them to contract.

If the muscles stay contracted due to intense exercise or if they stay flaccid due to lack of exercise, lymph circulation will decrease drastically inside muscles, and edema can result. This is particularly true as people age. Exercise is also beneficial because it moves the skin, which helps to open the flaps of the initial lymphatics, allowing more fluid to enter the lymphatic system.

Excessive Dietary Salt

The body maintains a specific salt-to-fluid ratio. The more salt a person consumes, the more water will be retained in the tissues to balance the salt. This water buildup will result in edema. Americans commonly eat food high in sodium, so this type of edema is common and usually temporary. It responds to massage and a decrease in the consumption of salt in the diet, as well as additional fluid intake. Besides high sodium, foods like strawberries and avocados, which are common allergens, can cause swelling.

Scar Tissue and Soft Tissue Injury

When tissue is damaged, blood and lymph vessels rupture. Lymph circulation is inhibited by vessel damage. As the injured area heals and scar tissue forms, lymph circulation does not always improve. Lymph vessels and blood vessels grow in the new scar tissue, but they do not necessarily connect to the lymph vessels on the other side of the scar. Scar tissue can result from injury, surgery, or infection. Edema tends to form on the side of the scarring distal to, or farthest from, the nodes. Small pockets of edema can remain for years in an injured area. Even if many years have elapsed after an injury and the accompanying edema has become chronic, the edema will respond to a combination of connective tissue massage and LDM.

Heart or Kidney Disease

Heart and kidney diseases affect fluid circulation in the body. When the heart or kidneys are diseased, their ability to handle fluid is compromised. There is inadequate force to pump fluid up from the extremities, so fluid can accumulate in the hands and arms, or feet and legs. Lymph massage stimulates the lymph circulation and returns fluid to the heart. As a result, blood volume increases, which, in the case of a person with heart disease, could overload an already weakened heart. Similarly, because the kidneys regulate blood volume, an increase in blood volume could overload already weakened kidneys.

Medication

Some medications contribute to edema, particularly steroids like cortisone and female hormone therapy. Chemotherapy for cancer can cause edema as a side effect.

Radiation Therapy

Radiation therapy scars the tissue through which it passes, causing obstructive edema. Lymph vessels in the area are damaged along with other tissues, so lymph flow is obstructed in a large area.

Allergies

Insect bites and other allergens stimulate the inflammatory response that causes swelling. Because insects sometimes inject poisons with the bite or sting, massage should not be performed in any swollen areas while symptoms are acute. Once symptoms subside and the area is no longer sensitive, massage is safe.

Menstrual Cycle

Water retention and/or a swollen abdomen and extremities are common before or during the menstrual cycle. Gentle lymph massage on the abdomen during menses is safe, but no deep massage should be performed.

Emotional Tension

Stress is infrequently recognized as a cause of edema, yet practitioners commonly observe that chronic tension due to stress contributes to edema in a specific area. For example, people suffering muscle-tension headaches often have palpable edema in the region of the occipital muscles due to spasm and inflammation of strained suboccipital muscles. With migraine headaches, elevated blood pressure in the cerebral arteries can produce edema in the tissues below the cranium.[4]

LYMPHEDEMA DISEASE

When edema becomes chronic, it is called lymphedema disease. Lymphedema disease progresses over time and, at the least, is uncomfortable and reduces the quality of life, impacting on daily activities. At the worst, lymphedema disease results in chronic serious infections. At this stage, it is painful and impacts seriously on the quality of life, making daily activities difficult, if not impossible.

Lymphedema disease is a progressive disorder that cannot be cured, although it does respond to LDM, bandaging, and exercise; comprehensive decongestive therapy consists of these three components when used together. Ideally, clients with lymphedema would be referred by their physicians to therapists with advanced training in these areas. A beginning lymph drainage massage therapist may want to work with more experienced therapists or under the direction of a physician before attempting to help people with more advanced cases of edema.

Review the contraindications with every client so as to avoid doing harm. If a client has lymphedema disease in the third or fourth stage (see the discussion on staging of lymphedema elsewhere in the text), any kind of massage should be given only under the physician's supervision.

Lymphedema disease is chronic and goes through different stages over time. Edema can feel soft and spongy, or very hard. At an early stage, edema can feel hard when fluid has filled the capacity of the skin, and the skin is stretching to contain the fluid. This feels smooth and hard to the touch, and is painful to the client. Early stages of edema may cause the pitting characteristic in skin.

To identify pitting, press a fingertip into the tissue, and then withdraw it. Any remaining indentation is called pitting edema. The indentation may fill quickly or remain visible for a while. Tissue can be tender when compressed, or painful because the swelling is pressing on nerves.

As time passes, the condition of the skin changes. There is not only an excess of tissue fluid, but also the growth of scar tissue in the skin and underlying structures. The stagnant tissue fluid contains proteins, microorganisms, and toxins. Microorganisms reproduce, causing infections. Protein buildup in tissues triggers inflammation. Part of the inflammatory process is the migration of connective tissue fibers to the area. Over time, the tissue changes in texture and appearance, becoming thicker, less flexible, reddened, and coarse. It feels cool to the touch unless there is an infection.

Edema is abnormal, so its presence indicates pathology of some sort, from temporary conditions caused by inactivity or minor injury, to serious illnesses such as heart or kidney disease. Edema that does not abate in a day or two should be evaluated by a physician to rule out serious health problems.

Edematous tissues have poor oxygenation, poor nutrition, poor waste removal, reduced function, and heal slowly after injury. Chronic inflammation and **fibrosis** make the edematous tissue coarser, thicker, less flexible, and more tender due to increased neurofibrils in the injury area.[5,6] When edema is present, it is difficult to palpate underlying structures such as muscles and bones.

Lymphedema can be diagnosed with a CT or MRI scan, **lymphangiography** or **lymphoscintigraphy**. However, these tests aren't always done. The diagnosis of lymphedema can be made if there is visibly swollen tissue in a patient who presents with complaints of pain, difficulty in movement, changes in the texture and temperature of the skin, and swelling that occurred following injury, infection, surgery, or some other incident that blocked the lymphatics or lymph nodes.

Lymphedema is different from obesity, in that obesity tends to be symmetrical but lymphedema is confined to the obstructed area. However, at later stages in lymphedema, there is a growth of fat cells in the lymphedematous tissue, complicating its appearance and further degrading the condition, making treatment more difficult.[7]

Treatment of lymphedema disease varies, but usually includes lymph drainage massage, compression with bandages or elastic sleeves, and range of motion exercises. Treatment also includes diligent skin care in order to prevent further injury, infection, and breakdown of the skin. Exercise should be designed to stimulate lymph drainage (stretching exercises, for instance) without making things worse through over-exertion.

For a healthy person without lymphedema disease, exercise is an important factor in lymph circulation. Gentle rebounding, walking, dancing, even yawning and stretching, tai chi, qigong and yoga all stimulate lymph circulation, from the opening of the initial lymphatics in the periphery of the body to the squeezing of the thoracic duct deep in the center of the body as a deep breath is taken.

For the person with lymphedema disease, exercise is just as important. However, the affected limb should not be injured during the process. He or she should wear compression garments while exercising to protect the affected limb and to inhibit swelling due to increased filtration from blood vessels into the tissues. Exercise significantly increases the flow of lymph through the thoracic duct, as well as improving strength, endurance, flexibility and range of motion. Exercise, performed while wearing compression garments and with adequate rest between sets, has been shown to increase lymph flow but doesn't worsen lymphedema disease.[8,9]

Primary Lymphedema

The cause of **primary lymphedema** is uncertain. In some cases, the cause of the lymphedema is known, including congenital abnormalities of large lymph vessels such as the thoracic duct, insufficient number of lymph vessels, lymph valves that don't function properly, or lymph node scarring. If the condition develops in the first few years of life, the cause is likely congenital. If the condition develops later in life, the cause may be a disease that destroys lymph vessels and/or nodes.[10]

For instance, there may be an abnormal abundance of blood vessels in one leg. In that case, the surplus blood vessels would release more tissue fluids into the tissues of the leg than the lymphatic system could absorb and carry away from the limb. This would cause chronic edema in the affected leg, while the other limb would remain normal. In another case, the cause of congenital lymphedema could be the lack of lymph vessels in an area. More women than men experience congenital lymphedema disease.

Secondary Lymphedema

Secondary lymphedema is caused by obstruction due to infection, injury, irradiation, or surgery. In Africa, for instance, **elephantiasis** is a very advanced form of lymphedema caused by a parasite that infects and scars the lymphatics. In more developed countries, lymphedema often follows cancer surgery if tissue and lymph nodes are surgically removed, causing scarring. Radiation therapy scars the tissues through which it passes, hardening those tissues as if they had been cooked.

Lymphedema disease has serious complications. Because of scar tissue, fluid is not removed from tissues normally. Instead, the fluid stays in the tissues and stagnates. Bacteria can multiply, causing cellulitis, a serious infection that is difficult to heal and can sometimes lead to amputation. Chronic lymphedema disease can cause the skin to thicken, cool, and coarsen and become prone to injury and infection. The body treats proteins in stagnant interstitial fluid as foreign particles, which cause inflammation and its symptoms of pain, heat, redness, and more edema.[11] Chronic inflammation creates a sort of feedback loop in which the inflammation causes tissues to scar, and scar tissue blocks lymph circulation. As the capacity of the lymphatic system becomes limited, blood vessels continue to release fluid into those tissues, increasing the edema. This causes stress on skin and connective tissue which causes more inflammation. The gross deformities of elephantiasis show how severe the problem can become.

Patients with lymphedema disease must scrupulously protect their edematous limbs from injury and infection. Chronic lymphedema disease is painful and disfiguring, and patients with lymphedema disease may struggle with depression because the disease limits their ability to move and function normally. A severe case can render a patient housebound and sedentary.

Working with Lymphedema

Clearly, working with lymphedema disease is a job for experienced practitioners who have had advanced training and some clinical practice. In clinical practice, under supervision, therapists are more aware of contraindications and the serious problems that might arise in treatment. They gain experience dealing with all the manifestations of lymphedema. Beginning LDM therapists should not be afraid to help anyone who comes to them, but should definitely work under the supervision of an experienced therapist or medical practitioner.

Stages of Lymphedema Disease

Stage 0 is the preclinical stage, with no visible evidence of lymph flow impedance. However, evaluation by means of bioimpedance, a diagnostic tool that shows the composition of body tissues, may show that lymph flow is compromised. Starting lymph drainage massage as soon as cancer surgery heals, and continuing during radiation therapy, can help prevent lymphedema.

In stage 1 lymphedema, there is visible swelling, tissue is soft and there may be pitting edema. The swelling responds to elevation of the limb, and to massage. Comprehensive decongestive therapy begun at this stage may control the edema and prevent it from becoming more severe.

In stage 2 lymphedema, tissues begin to change, becoming increasingly firm due to fibrosis. The edema no longer responds to elevation and massage only produces temporary improvement. At this stage, more intense treatment is required. Connective tissue massage may be needed in addition to lymph drainage massage and comprehensive decongestive therapy. The condition may be increasingly painful and there may be difficulty in accomplishing normal daily activities.

In stage 3 lymphedema, the tissue becomes extremely swollen, hardened, loses elasticity and changes color. Daily functions are very difficult and quality of life diminishes due to pain, disfigurement, lack of mobility, repeated infections and open wounds. Because of the infections and compromised skin integrity, lymph massage should only be performed under the direction of a physician.[12]

Occasionally, surgery is performed to remove abnormal tissue. However, this surgery itself creates scar tissue and has had limited success. Lymphedema disease is a lifelong condition and clients/patients have to be diligent about massage, proper exercise, and scrupulous skin care.[13]

REVIEW QUESTIONS

1. How does dietary salt intake contribute to edema?
2. What are the common causes of obstructive edema?
3. How does exercise affect lymph circulation in muscles?
4. Besides obstruction, what other factors may contribute to edema?
5. Describe pitting edema.
6. What tissue changes occur with chronic edema?
7. What is the long-term outlook for lymphedema disease?
8. What are the possible complications of chronic lymphedema disease?
9. How is lymphedema disease treated?
10. What factors can cause edema?
11. What is primary lymphedema?
12. What is secondary lymphedema?
13. What factors or events can cause obstructive lymphedema?
14. Describe some complications of lymphedema.

Lymph Drainage Massage: Indications and Contraindications

L ymph drainage massage is a valuable technique for many kinds of practitioners. Although it is usually associated with the medical treatment of lymphedema, LDM can be used for many different conditions, and benefits healthy people as much as it benefits people with serious illnesses.

While LDM is very gentle and safe, it stimulates physiological changes in the body and should not be used in some instances. Therapists should be familiar with LDM contraindications and should be able to explain the reasons for the contraindications to their clients. It may be necessary to deny a massage to some clients because of health conditions that would be exacerbated by the massage. In some cases, therapists can modify the massage to avoid injuring a client.

INDICATIONS

Lymph drainage massage has many benefits. It stimulates the circulation of lymph and blood, and moves tissue fluid from the tissues into lymph vessels. Lymph vessels carry lymph and its contents through the lymph nodes, where the fluid is purified. Eventually, purified lymphatic fluid is returned to blood circulation.

In this process, toxins such as microorganisms, microscopic particles, metabolic waste, and chemicals are removed from tissues. Proteins are also removed from tissues and are returned to blood circulation, preventing protein buildup in the tissues, which leads to chronic inflammation.

Increased lymph flow helps to distribute immune cells throughout the body, reducing infection and speeding the healing of inflammation.

Because LDM is relaxing, nurturing, and supporting, it helps decrease stress, depression, insomnia, and fatigue. Removing edema and relaxing soft tissues, including muscles, reduces pain.

Deep abdominal lymph massage reduces constipation and abdominal pain, helps to restore intestinal peristalsis, relaxes adhesions in the abdomen, improves the motility of abdominal organs, and improves breathing. All of these help to stimulate the deep circulation of lymph.

MORE INDICATIONS FOR LDM

Edema

Lymph drainage massage is very effective in reducing edema. However, it is important to know the cause of the edema before proceeding. Edema can be a simple problem due to inactivity, hormonal changes, diet, or scar tissue. Scar tissue can result from injuries, surgery, radiation, or infections. Edema is sometimes a side effect of medical treatment, such as treatment with steroids.

Edema can be a symptom of more serious conditions that can be aggravated by massage. Anyone who has chronic edema and does not know the cause should consult a physician to rule out serious health problems before receiving LDM.

Surgery

LDM may be used before and after surgery, including cosmetic surgery, to speed healing and reduce edema. Before surgery, LDM helps to remove stagnant fluid from tissues and increase blood flow, which brings nutrition to the tissues. LDM is also deeply relaxing, so it can lessen the client's stress and anxiety. Because the massage is so deeply relaxing, in fact, somewhat hypnotic, the therapist can help clients by listening to their feelings about the surgery and by making positive statements about the outcome. One of the most beneficial effects of massage in a medical setting is that it meets the clients' needs for support and nurturing, which physicians and families cannot always provide.

After surgery, LDM can help to remove inflammation, speed healing, and reduce scar tissue. Because of the risk of infection and the risk of blood clots, LDM should never be performed immediately after surgery without the approval, and possibly the direction, of the client's physician. It is usually necessary to delay massage until the physician releases the client and the client needs no more medical treatment, at which time the client will have healed completely and massage is likely to be safe.

Soft Tissue Injury

In the case of soft tissue injury, LDM speeds healing and reduces swelling. For minor injuries that are healing, massage is safe. During the acute phase of the injury, lymph drainage massage can begin draining the swelling around the injured area, reducing scarring, and removing metabolic waste. Serious injuries should be examined by a doctor before massage to rule out any serious underlying damage which could be exacerbated by massage. A good rule of thumb is to have the client evaluate the amount of pain he or she is experiencing, and whether the injury is healing and the pain decreasing. If pain is severe, or if pain is increasing rather than decreasing as time passes, a massage therapist should refer the client to a physician for evaluation. After appropriate medical treatment, LDM helps to speed healing, reduce inflammation and pain, and improve scars.

Sluggish Immune System

Frequent colds and allergies are indications for LDM. Healthy adults should be able to resist most mild illnesses to which they are exposed. If a client is frequently ill with minor illnesses and recovers slowly, and a medical evaluation hasn't uncovered any serious health problem, the immune system may be sluggish. In that case, LDM will stimulate the circulation of white blood cells through the lymphatic system and potentially improve the condition. Encourage a client who is frequently ill with minor illnesses to have LDM regularly, daily, if possible, for a week, or at least once a week for three months. In fact, it was for this kind of condition that Dr. Vodder originally developed lymph drainage massage.

Relieving Stress and Tension

Stress triggers the sympathetic nervous system, the well-known fight-or-flight state, arousing all the body's defenses. Chemicals like adrenaline are secreted into the bloodstream, causing muscles to tense. Heart and respiratory rates increase, organ function decreases, and the immune system is suppressed. Chronic stress results in chronic "racing" of the human system, with resulting stress on internal organs and functions and decreased disease resistance. In the long run, physical and mental reactions to stress can contribute to degenerative disease. Massage, and especially LDM, trigger the parasympathetic nervous system, which has the opposite effect on the body. Muscles relax, heart and breathing rates decrease, and clients move into a drowsy state of relaxation that promotes healing and balance.

Fatigue, Mild Depression, and Chronic Soft Tissue Pain

Symptoms like fatigue, mild depression, and chronic soft tissue pain call for the gentleness of lymph massage. It is important for a person who has these symptoms and does not know the cause to have a physical examination by a physician, an acupuncturist, or another licensed healthcare provider to rule out serious health problems. If no serious illness underlying the symptoms can be discovered, LDM can be given with good results; it will stimulate the immune system and has an energizing effect on the body's *qi* or vital energy.

Working with Positional Edema

Enforced inactivity, such as sitting in an airplane, in a car, or at a desk for several hours at a time, causes edema. If the legs remain still for long periods of time, the calf muscles won't contract, which normally helps blood and fluids circulate. The force of gravity pulling down the interstitial fluids will be stronger than the forces pulling up the fluids. This can cause swelling in the feet, hands, and buttocks of a person who has to sit for a few hours. Lymph drainage massage drains excess tissue fluid and reduces the pain and stiffness that accompany the swelling.

There is a risk of a blood clot, also called deep vein thrombosis, when someone has been sitting still for a long time and also has risk factors present for conditions that would slow or change the flow of blood in the veins. These include medications such as estrogen or birth control pills, obesity, pregnancy, cancer, recent surgery or fractures, cigarette smoking, a pacemaker or a heart condition, or a blood-clotting disorder. If your client has pain in the calf and the calf is red, hot, swollen, and painful, there may be a blood clot. Do *not* massage. Instead, refer the client to his or her physician *immediately* for diagnosis and treatment.

Diet

An excess of salty food causes the body to retain water, resulting in edema. The human organism maintains a specific ratio of fluid to salts. Eating a high-salt diet leads to edema, as the body retains enough fluid to balance the salt. LDM can remove excess fluid from tissues, and return the fluid to the bloodstream for excretion through the kidneys. Encourage the client to drink more water to wash salt out of the body through the kidneys, and to reduce dietary salt intake in order to avoid having the problem occur again.

Scar Tissue

Scar tissue obstructs lymph flow. Lymph vessels damaged by injury or surgery are scarred, and lymph flow is hindered. New lymph vessels may not grow through the scar tissue in an organized way to connect to lymph circulation on the other side of the scar. The obstruction of lymph flow leads to an accumulation of fluid in tissues around the scar.

LDM reduces edema and also softens and minimizes scars, improving circulation. One of the effects of LDM is to move tissue fluid around obstructions, toward areas with less tissue fluid, and from there into unobstructed lymph vessels. Massaging as soon as allowable after an injury or surgery actually helps scars to develop in a more organized way so that they are smaller, smoother, and more flexible than scar tissue that hasn't had the benefit of massage.

Enhancing the Skin

Unhealthy skin caused by poor circulation improves with LDM. The massage removes wastes and toxins from skin cells and stimulates blood circulation, bringing nutrients to the skin. This is particularly useful in esthetics. LDM helps such conditions as acne, rosacea, and eczema. Avoid massage during the acute phase of any skin condition.

LDM benefits the red, thickened, coarse skin that results from chronic edema and that is common in the lower extremities of clients with lymphedema, and in clients who are obese. However, do not massage any area that is infected or inflamed (red, hot, swollen, and painful), as this could spread infectious microorganisms beyond the infected area into tissue that is not infected. Massage should be delayed until the condition has been treated and is beginning to improve.

CONTRAINDICATIONS

Although LDM is very beneficial and safe for most people, some conditions may be exacerbated by massage. Some contraindications are absolute, but some merely require that the therapist take precautions or consult with the client's physician before performing the massage.

Thrombosis and Phlebitis

Blood clots and **phlebitis** are contraindications for any kind of massage. Blood clots are possible during the first 2 weeks following surgery or injury, and massage can cause a blood clot to break loose and move through the circulatory system to the lungs or heart. Such an occurrence is potentially life-threatening. It is best to avoid massage entirely for 2 weeks after surgery, unless the client's physician deems it safe.

If a client has a history of phlebitis, which is inflammation of the walls of a vein, or is taking blood-thinning medication, such as Coumadin (Warfarin), consult the client's physician before giving a massage. Closely examine varicose veins before massaging the area. If the area with varicose veins is warmer than the surrounding tissue, or reddened, swollen, and painful, do not give massage. An area with spider veins and protruding veins that are not red, hot, swollen, and painful may be massaged carefully. The very light pressure of LDM is safe as long as the veins are asymptomatic.

Risk Factors for Blood Clot (Embolism)

- major surgery under general anesthesia
- obesity
- varicose veins
- prolonged immobility
- major injuries
- cancer
- pregnancy and childbirth
- estrogen containing contraceptive pills, patch, or vaginal ring
- estrogen replacement therapy
- long-distance travel

Serious Illness

The simplest and safest procedure to follow in working with clients with serious illnesses is to ask these clients to bring a signed, written statement from their doctors affirming that massage is not likely to harm the client. When working with clients who have serious illness, it's important for the massage therapist to see himself or herself as part of the client's healthcare team. Members of the healthcare team have to work together to support the client's well-being and to avoid harm. When the client is being treated for a serious illness, the physician and client are in charge of health treatment decisions, not the massage therapist. It's important for the physician to know that the client is receiving massage to avoid the possibility of exacerbating the condition or interfering with the client's medical treatment.

Traditionally, massage has been contraindicated for patients with active cancer for fear of causing the cancer to metastasize. However, there is no compelling evidence that LDM is dangerous for cancer patients. In fact, a client's physician may feel that the benefits from touch therapy outweigh the risks and thus recommend massage, including lymph massage.[1] The decision whether to give LDM to a person with active cancer should not be made independently. When clients are very ill and receiving medical treatment, the massage therapist should consult with the clients' healthcare providers before giving the massage. This is especially true when clients are taking chemotherapy for the treatment of cancer. It is usually safe and beneficial to give LDM to a client who is undergoing radiation treatment. When a client is in remission and no longer being treated for cancer, LDM is generally considered safe.

If major organs in the body, such as the heart, kidneys, or liver, are damaged and unable to function normally, edema may occur. However, even though edema is present, LDM is not appropriate in these cases. LDM returns fluid to the cardiovascular system, increasing blood volume. A weak heart may be unable to handle the increased load, stressing the heart. The kidneys control blood volume by excreting excess fluid. If the kidneys are failing, the increased volume of fluid in the blood can be too stressful. Give LDM to no one who has had a heart attack or heart surgery in the previous year, who is experiencing congestive heart failure or kidney failure, or who is undergoing kidney dialysis. If the client has liver disease, consult with the client's physician before giving massage.[2]

Acute Conditions and Infectious Conditions

Avoid massage during the acute phase of an illness. Allow the lymphatic system to handle the illness at its own pace. Do not massage a client who has a contagious condition. Therapists want to prevent spreading contagion to themselves, their families, and other clients.

Avoid giving massage to a person with a fever. Fever is part of the body's natural healing process. When fever is present, white blood cells circulate more quickly and reproduce more quickly so that they can defeat disease-producing microorganisms. Massage tends to normalize body functions, and can lower the client's temperature, defeating the purpose of a fever. It is important for the therapist's health, as well, to deny massage to a client with a fever, to avoid contagion. Encourage a client with a fever to rest and recover.

Inflammation (redness, swelling, heat, and pain) in any area of the body is a sign of injury, illness, or infection. Determine the cause of the inflammation before proceeding. In the case of chronic infections, massage may cause a flare-up of the infection, worsening the condition. Check with the client's physician before giving a massage.

Massage, including LDM, is contraindicated for any skin condition that is contagious, infected, open, discharging fluid, or inflamed (red, hot, swollen, or painful).

Asthma

LDM may trigger an asthma attack in those with severe asthma. Do not give LDM during or following an asthma attack. If the client has a history of being hospitalized with asthma, or is on daily asthma medication, give very short sessions until tolerance is determined.

Allergies

Allergic symptoms result from an overreaction of the immune system to allergens. Do not give LDM during an allergic reaction, as this stimulates lymph circulation and immune function and can spread histamines, which could result in increased inflammation. After the client has recovered from acute allergic symptoms, it is safe to proceed with LDM. Regular LDM to the face and neck helps to reduce chronic sinus infections and allergies.

Thyroid

It is possible to aggravate hyperthyroidism by massaging over the area of the thyroid. For clients with thyroid disease, any style of massage is contraindicated for the area where the thyroid is located, which is the front of the neck between the two sternocleidomastoid muscles. Because Graves' disease and Hashimoto's disease are autoimmune disorders, it is also contraindicated for the lymph nodes medial to the sternocleidomastoid muscles.[3,4]

Low Blood Pressure

Take care with clients who have low blood pressure. LDM lowers blood pressure, so there is the danger that clients with low blood pressure may become dizzy or faint upon standing after a massage. Avoid lengthy sessions, and be sure clients are awake and feeling fine before standing. Sitting on the massage table with the legs dangling for a few minutes before standing will reduce the risk of fainting.

INTAKE FORM

Use an intake form to save time and keep a written record of the session. After reviewing the intake form, the therapist may wish to ask additional questions and should take note of the client's answers. Following is a detailed list of questions to ask your clients.

What is your primary reason for this visit?

What do you want to accomplish with this session?

What other areas need attention?

Are you currently experiencing a cold, flu, inflammation, fever, infection, or other condition that may be contagious?

Medications (check all that apply)

- Heart medicines
- Blood pressure medicine
- Blood thinner
- Painkillers
- Cortisone injection, steroid medication
- Anti-inflammatory medication
- Muscle relaxant

Musculoskeletal symptoms (check all that apply)

- Fibromyalgia or similar conditions
- Spasm, cramps, sprains, strains
- Osteoporosis
- Scoliosis, lordosis or kyphosis
- Whiplash, torticollis, other neck pain
- Tendonitis, carpal tunnel syndrome, sciatica, thoracic outlet syndrome, plantar fasciitis
- Joint problems (for example, bursitis, osteoarthritis, rheumatoid arthritis, gout, recent dislocation, sprain)
- Spinal injury
- Fracture
- Bone cancer

Skin conditions (check all that apply)

- Infectious conditions such as acne, fungus, impetigo, open wound or sore, athlete's foot, rash
- Eczema, psoriasis, dermatitis
- Skin cancer
- Warts, moles, scars
- Swelling, redness, heat, pain, bruise

Cardiovascular disease (check all that apply)

- Congestive heart failure, heart attack, heart surgery, arrhythmia, high or low blood pressure
- Blood clot, phlebitis, varicose veins, stroke, deep vein thrombosis, embolism
- Arteriosclerosis
- Anemia

Other (check all that apply)

- Liver disease, liver failure
- Kidney disease, kidney failure, bladder conditions, urinary tract infections
- Diabetes, Syndrome X (metabolic syndrome)

Neurological conditions (check all that apply)

- Numbness or tingling in any area of the body
- Damage from stroke
- Epilepsy
- Multiple sclerosis
- Cerebral palsy

More

- Recent accident, injury, or surgery (for example, a fall, auto accident, whiplash, sprain, broken bone, deep bruise, dental surgery, outpatient surgery, in-hospital surgery). Are any of these conditions still affecting you now?
- Lymphatic system condition (for example, swollen nodes, edema, any disease of the lymphatic system)
- Digestive system conditions (for example, ulcers, heartburn, hiatal hernia, colitis, irritable bowel)
- Immune system conditions (for example, HIV/AIDS, autoimmune disease)
- Headaches

Site restrictions

Are there any areas of your body that should be avoided by the massage therapist?

- Incisions, open wounds, drains, dressings
- IV port, ostomy, catheter, or other device
- Radiation site, or site of a tumor, skin tumor
- Skin sensitivity, rash, or skin condition
- Neuropathy
- Injury
- Area of infection
- Are there any other areas that should be avoided?

Please describe:_____

Pressure restrictions

Are there any areas where pressure should be avoided during the massage?

- Lymphedema disease
- Tender or painful areas
- Bruising or other injured area
- Sensitive skin, or scar tissue

Please describe:_____

Position restriction

Are there any positions that you cannot tolerate?

Please describe: _____

What is the cause?

- Incisions, open wounds, drains, dressings
- Dizziness
- Ostomy bag or other medical device
- Tumor site
- Difficulty breathing (note in which positions)
- Injured or swollen limb that should be elevated
- Discomfort
- Pregnancy
- Other

Cancer

What is the diagnosis? When were you diagnosed?

Where was/is it located?

Did you have surgery? When? What kind of surgery?

What other treatment did you receive? (for example, chemotherapy or radiation, lymph node removal)

What is your current condition?

Are you still being treated now?

What was the date of your last treatment?

Pain

Are you currently experiencing pain?

Where? Do you know the cause?

Can you describe it?

When did the pain first appear?

Is it constant or intermittent? How long does it last?

Does it move—different locations at different times?

Is the pain sharp or dull?

What makes your pain better?

- Heat
- Pressure
- Movement
- Cold
- Massage
- Rest

Describe anything else which makes your pain better _____

What makes your pain worse?

- Activity
- Exercise
- Certain positions
- Heat or cold

Is there anything else that makes the pain worse?

_____

Are you taking any medications to control the pain?

Are you using home remedies such as heat or ice to control the pain?

ACTIVITIES

1. Using the sample questions above and searching for sample intake forms on the Internet, create your own custom intake form for your clients.

2. Create a SOAP (Subjective Objective Assessment Plan) form to use after every session. It should include a space for the date, the therapist's name, type of massage given, any additional information the client reveals about his or her condition, results of the previous session, and recommendations or referrals made by the therapist. If more than one therapist is likely to work on the client over a period of time, make sure to include information that the next therapist will need to know.

Principles of Lymph Drainage Massage

L ymph drainage massage is perhaps the most researched and scientifically validated form of massage in the world. A significant body of scientific evidence supports the effectiveness of massage in reducing edema.[1,2,3,4,5]

Although LDM may seem labor-intensive, complicated and time-consuming, modern evidence indicates that success depends on only a few necessary principles, and in fact, simple self-treatment procedures can effectively move lymph.[6]

LYMPH DRAINAGE MASSAGE PRINCIPLES

Lymph drainage massage involves more than moving tissue fluid into the initial lymphatics, and out of the skin, muscles, and organs. Peripheral lymphatics are embedded in the fascia, or connective tissue, and in the tissue fluid, a gel-like liquid tissue. Lymph massage includes relaxing the connective tissue, warming tissue fluid so that it flows more easily, moving tissue fluid out of intercellular spaces and into the initial lymphatics, pumping lymph fluid toward the lymph nodes, and stimulating lymph vessels to contract on their own by mimicking the workings of the lymphatic vessels.

When moving lymph fluid, certain principles are more meaningful than specific hand movements. The greatest success in reducing edema and stimulating lymph circulation results when these principles are followed. Massage techniques that do not conform to these principles do not move lymph as efficiently, although they are still beneficial.

When first learning LDM, it helps to have an instructor demonstrate exactly where to place the hands, and for how long to massage each area. With experience, the therapist will progress from following a detailed outline to more intuitive work, correctly responding to tissue changes that indicate the therapy has succeeded.

Clients who are accustomed to receiving full-body massages in one hour may be surprised to find that this cannot be done with lymph drainage massage. Because the massage is very slow, it can take up to an hour to massage one quadrant of the trunk and the limb connected to it.

Reducing lymph stasis, or stagnation, takes more time than would be involved in moving lymph in an area with no obstruction. It may take several sessions over just one quadrant of the body to reduce edema when there is obstruction. If the client has no edema and is in reasonably good health, lymph will move more quickly and the massage will take less time, allowing the therapist to cover a larger area.

Palpation

Lymph nodes are small and bean-shaped. Normally, it is difficult to palpate lymph nodes because they are soft and not tender, except in the presence of infection, inflammation or tumor growth. An enlarged, scarred or inflamed lymph node feels like a small bean beneath the skin. It moves with the skin, not with the muscles, and is more superficial than skeletal muscles. Using knowledge of lymph anatomy, the therapist or esthetician palpates in the areas where lymph nodes can be found. If lymph nodes can be felt, they may be full of white blood cells responding to attack, or they may be scarred due to previous infection and inflammation. They may also be enlarged due to tumor growth. If nodes can be identified by palpation, ask the client whether he or she has ever had them examined by a doctor. If not, then recommend that the client do so at the next visit to a physician.

Edema and fat feel similar, but with practice, it is possible to learn to palpate the difference between the two. Fat is generally symmetrical, appearing the same on the right and left sides of the body, and above and below the waist. Edema is generally not symmetrical. Edema is located in the superficial tissues as well as the muscles below. Fibrosis, the deposit of fibers in tissues, is inflexible and tender. It can be distinguished from muscle tissue because muscle fibers are aligned in a specific direction, while fibrosis is more irregular than muscle tissues and feels coarser.

Move the Skin

There is a rich bed of lymph capillaries in the superficial tissues, close to the surface of the skin, and edema occurs in these superficial tissues more often than in deep tissue. LDM focuses on this bed of lymph capillaries. Success depends on moving the skin. Stretching the skin lengthwise, horizontally, and diagonally stretches the initial lymphatics and lymph capillaries, stimulating them to contract.[7]

Moving the skin also pulls the microfilaments that connect the initial lymphatics to the surrounding tissues, causing the endothelial flaps to open and allowing interstitial fluid to enter the initial lymphatics. Lymphatic capillaries are located in a fiber matrix, the fascia, and are surrounded by intercellular fluid, which is somewhat like a gel at rest. Stretching the skin gently in a circle helps to warm tissue fluid, causing it to move more freely.

Stretching the skin also helps relax the connective tissue, or fascia, which supports and contains lymphatic capillaries. Chronic edema causes chronic inflammation, which causes tissue to thicken and become coarser. This makes the connective tissue less supple and less flexible, which inhibits lymph circulation. Moving the skin gently in the process of lymph drainage massage has an effect similar to myofascial release—it gently relaxes and stretches connective tissue.

Apply Gentle Pressure

A light pressure must be used to massage severe edema in soft tissue. Vodder estimated the proper pressure for lymph drainage to be less than 30 torr, or 9 ounces per square inch.[8,9] This figure is very close to what Zweifach and Prather obtained after sampling lymphatic pressures in 1975. The pressure in the peripheral lymphatics is even less, approximately one half ounce to eight ounces per square inch.[10]

Therefore, the most effective pressure for lymph drainage massage is between one half ounce and eight ounces per square inch. At the beginning of the massage, the pressure should be as light as possible, while still moving the skin. As the massage progresses and the therapist feels changes in the tissue which indicate that the lymph is beginning to drain out of the area, the pressure can increase, becoming closer to eight ounces per square inch. To strive for accuracy, it helps to practice by stroking the surface of a postage scale until one can easily keep the pressure in the recommended range.

Deep massage is contraindicated over areas of lymphedema. Deep pressure is more likely to damage lymph vessels where there is lymphedema than where tissue is normal, and more time will be required for lymph vessels to return to normal with deep pressure than if light pressure were used.[11,12]

Move Slowly

The greater the inertial mass (the amount of fluid in the tissue to be moved), the slower the movements must be. When there is a great deal of fluid to be moved, massage strokes may be repeated as slowly as six circles per minute, approximately the rate at which the peripheral lymphatics contract.[13] The rate of lymph flow is relatively slow compared to blood flow, but lymph flow is variable and can change, depending on outside influences. Therefore, LDM must be correspondingly slow, synchronizing with physiological processes. As the therapist begins to feel tissue change, the movements can be relatively faster, up to ten repetitions per minute.

Direction

Move lymph toward the lymph nodes in the neck, axilla, and groin. The lymph vessels effectively divide the body into four sections, excluding the head and neck. Each section consists of a limb and the adjacent quadrant of the trunk. The four quadrants are the:

1. Right arm and the upper-right quadrant of the trunk.
2. Left arm and the upper-left quadrant of the trunk.
3. Right leg and the lower-right quadrant of the trunk.
4. Left leg and the lower-left quadrant of the trunk.

The basic pattern of massage is to drain the lymph nodes first, and then the adjacent quadrant of the trunk. After massaging the trunk quadrant, massage the extremity, proximal to distal, and then go back again to the area of the nodes. The purpose of massaging the lymph nodes first is to make room for more fluid, which will be drained from the adjacent areas. Lymph circulation slows at the lymph nodes, as discussed in the chapter on lymph circulation, and if a therapist starts massaging at the distal end of the limb and works toward the lymph nodes, without first draining the lymph nodes, fluid tends to accumulate in the tissues surrounding the lymph nodes, causing swelling and discomfort.[14]

Rhythm and Repetition

Smooth, rhythmic movements are essential for success. One effect of lymph drainage massage is that it coordinates the contractions of the lymphatics, which can be erratic. Slow, rhythmic repetition of massage movements stimulates a wave in the lymph fluid, similar to intestinal peristalsis.[15] Maintain connection with the same area of the skin for at least a minute, repeating the stroke with the same pressure, direction, and speed until there is a palpable change in the tissue.

LYMPH DRAINAGE PATTERNS

Understanding the direction in which lymph drains is vital for the success of LDM. The basic pattern of LDM follows the direction of lymph flow from the extremities and **watersheds** to the cervical, axillary, and inguinal nodes (Figure 8–1a and b). The lymph vessels resemble four large branching trees made up of lymph capillaries and vessels. The lymph vessels drain fluid from the outermost reaches of the trees (the watersheds and the extremities) toward the **axillary** and inguinal nodes (tree trunks) and, from the nodes, lymph vessels

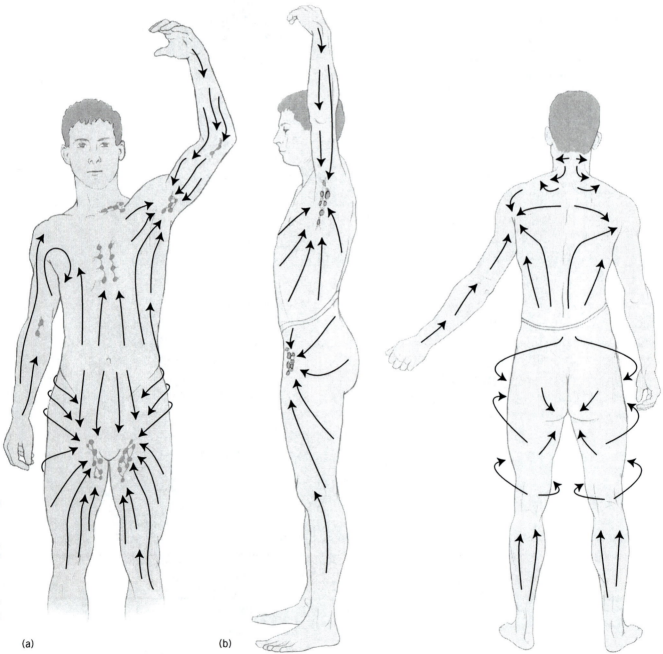

(a)   (b)

FIGURE 8–1a and b Direction of Lymph Flow

leading to the interior body are like the roots. At the watersheds, the branches of the trees overlap, but the drainage pattern is clearly demarcated.

Quadrants

Upper Body

In the upper body, between the waist and the clavicle, the peripheral lymphatics drain to the axillary lymph nodes. The right arm and right side of the trunk (anterior and posterior) drain toward the right axillary nodes. The left arm and the left side of the trunk drain toward the left axillary nodes. However, the lymphatics over the sternum drain upward to the **cervical nodes**, rather than toward the axillary nodes (Figure 8–2).

Lower Body

In the lower body, peripheral lymphatics drain to the inguinal nodes. The lymphatic vessels take the shortest route, so the superficial lymphatics in the buttocks drain laterally around the body to the inguinal nodes in front. The lymphatics in the posterior thigh divide—the lateral (outside) area of the thigh drains laterally around the leg, and the medial (inside) area of the thigh drains medially around the leg to the inguinal nodes. Lymph from the right leg and right lower quadrant of the trunk drains into the right inguinal nodes. Lymph from the left leg and the left lower quadrant of the trunk drains into the left inguinal nodes (Figure 8–3).

Executing Face and Neck Patterns

Lymph from the superficial lymphatics of the head drains inferiorly toward the lymph nodes in the neck. Lymph from the top of the head and the back of the head drains to the occipital nodes, and then toward the superior deep cervical nodes in the general area of the sternocleidomastoid muscle. Lymph from the facial lymphatics drains toward the preauricular and mandibular nodes, and then into the submandibular nodes before connecting to the superior deep cervical nodes (Figure 8–4).

Identifying Watersheds

The term "watershed" is used to refer to the four quadrants of drainage on the trunk, or the margins of the drainage areas. The direction of lymph drainage in the four trunk quadrants is not exact. Lymph capillaries form a network over the whole body, and the drainage of lymph in the four trunk quadrants is interconnected (Figure 8–5). In each area, most of the lymphatics drain toward the nearest nodes. However, some lymph capillaries, especially along the margins of the watershed areas, drain to adjacent quadrants. Around the waist, for instance, some lymph capillaries drain upward to the

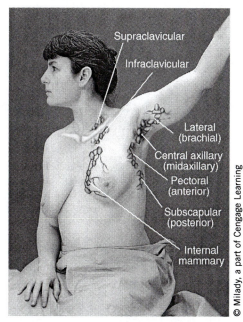

FIGURE 8-2 Upper quadrant and limb

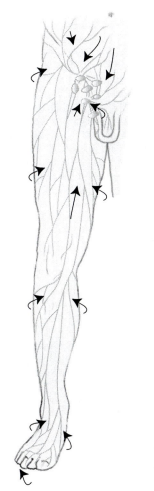

FIGURE 8-3 Lower quadrant and limb

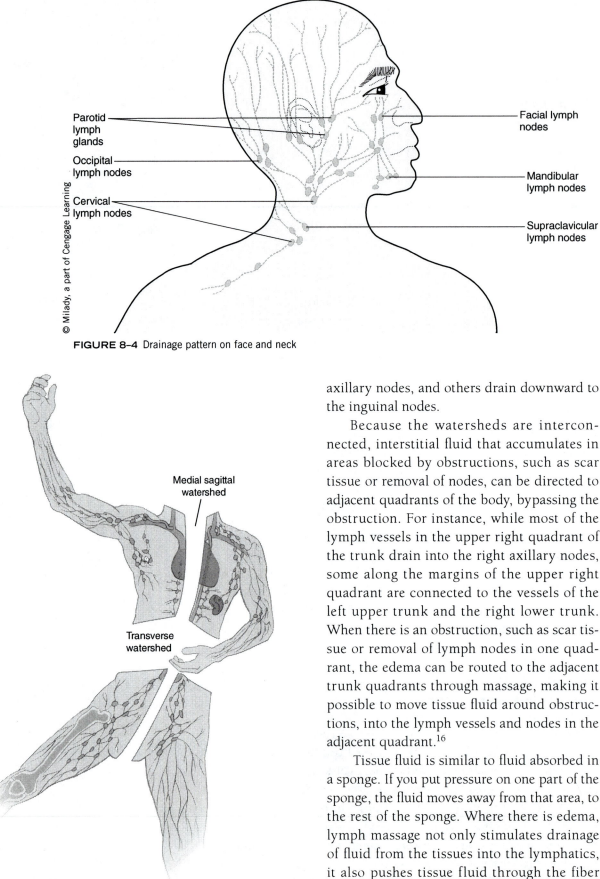

Parotid lymph glands

Occipital lymph nodes

Cervical lymph nodes

Facial lymph nodes

Mandibular lymph nodes

Supraclavicular lymph nodes

© Milady, a part of Cengage Learning

FIGURE 8–4 Drainage pattern on face and neck

Medial sagittal watershed

Transverse watershed

© Milady, a part of Cengage Learning

FIGURE 8–5 Watersheds

axillary nodes, and others drain downward to the inguinal nodes.

Because the watersheds are interconnected, interstitial fluid that accumulates in areas blocked by obstructions, such as scar tissue or removal of nodes, can be directed to adjacent quadrants of the body, bypassing the obstruction. For instance, while most of the lymph vessels in the upper right quadrant of the trunk drain into the right axillary nodes, some along the margins of the upper right quadrant are connected to the vessels of the left upper trunk and the right lower trunk. When there is an obstruction, such as scar tissue or removal of lymph nodes in one quadrant, the edema can be routed to the adjacent trunk quadrants through massage, making it possible to move tissue fluid around obstructions, into the lymph vessels and nodes in the adjacent quadrant.[16]

Tissue fluid is similar to fluid absorbed in a sponge. If you put pressure on one part of the sponge, the fluid moves away from that area, to the rest of the sponge. Where there is edema, lymph massage not only stimulates drainage of fluid from the tissues into the lymphatics, it also pushes tissue fluid through the fiber matrix to other areas nearby which are not as congested. The force of tissue fluid finding its way between cells from congested areas to areas with less pressure forms channels between cells, resembling the way channels form in the desert sand when there is a rainstorm. When rain falls so fast that the ground cannot absorb it all, the water will find its own way toward streams and creeks by making little channels through the sand.

MASSAGE SEQUENCE

For minor edema, begin the massage session by draining the lymph nodes of the affected quadrant. Because lymph drainage slows at the lymph nodes, the nodes must be drained first to make room for fluid drained from surrounding areas. Then, massage adjacent areas, moving fluid that is in the tissues near the lymph nodes into the lymph nodes themselves. Massage the adjacent trunk quadrant, working the lymph fluid toward the nodes.

Next, massage the affected limb proximal to distal, which means gradually working from the areas adjacent to the nodes out toward the distal end of the extremity. For example, if working on a swollen ankle, the therapist would first empty the inguinal nodes that are on the same side of the body as the swollen ankle. Next, she would massage the lower abdomen and buttocks on the same side as the affected ankle. Then she would massage the thigh (beginning close to the inguinal lymph nodes), the knee, and the lower limb (beginning at the knee and moving toward the ankle), gradually emptying the lymphatic vessels in the areas between the inguinal nodes and the edema. Finally, the therapist would massage the edematous ankle area itself, then work back up to the inguinal lymph nodes, emptying the inguinal nodes again at the end of the session. Depending on the degree of edema, the therapist may need to repeat the procedure until she feels a definite change in the edematous tissue.

For more serious conditions of obstructive edema, such as chronic swelling due to scar tissue from surgery, injury, or radiation, the general procedure is to massage the well side first, then the obstructed side. Following are the basic steps:

1. Massage the lymph nodes on the affected and unaffected sides of the body, including the inguinal, axillary, and cervical nodes.
2. Massage the trunk quadrant on the well side first. For instance, if the left arm is edematous, perform LDM on the upper-right quadrant of the trunk and/or the lower-left quadrant first.
3. Massage the trunk quadrant on the edematous side. In our example of the edematous left arm, this would be the upper-left quadrant of the trunk, closest to the area of lymph stasis.
4. Massage the proximal area of the edematous limb. In this case, that would be the upper-left arm, beginning at the shoulder, moving toward the elbow.
5. Massage the distal area of the edematous limb. In this case, that would be the lower-left arm, from the elbow toward the hand.

If the work has been performed carefully and slowly, by the time the therapist massages the entire extremity, the lymph should be moving more freely, and the lymphatic vessels should be contracting rhythmically. The therapist would then massage back toward the lymph nodes, away from the hand, moving with relatively more pressure and speed. The therapist would finish by massaging the lymph nodes again, then follow with closing strokes of the therapist's choosing, such as effleurage (which is described below).

MASSAGE MOVEMENTS

A wide variety of movements are taught in LDM. As long as therapists follow basic principles, any movement, whether circular, J-shaped, semicircular, or other, will work.

Stationary Circle

The basis of all LDM is the stationary circle. The **stationary circle** has two important components: (1) a slight compression and twist at the beginning of the movement and (2) a stretch of the tissues toward the lymph nodes. This move is called the stationary circle because it is important to remain stationary and repeat the movement six to ten times before moving to adjacent areas.

Using flat fingers, gently contact the skin, compress slightly, and twist the skin in a circular movement, stretching it toward the lymph nodes. Lighten the pressure and ride the skin back around to the starting point (Figure 8–6). Lymphatic capillaries are very close to the surface of the skin, so there is no need for deep pressure. The circular movement will stretch the lymph capillaries in different directions, stimulating them to contract. Also, gentle stationary circles cause the initial lymphatics to open, allowing interstitial fluid to enter through the endothelial flaps.

Pump

The pump is used on the extremities. Place the thumb on one side of the limb and wrap the palm and flat fingers around to the opposite side. Then, gently compress and stretch the skin with a scooping motion toward the appropriate lymph nodes, releasing pressure at the end of the movement (Figure 8–7). Repeat the pump movement until there is a palpable change in the skin.

"J" Strokes

To execute the "J" stroke, use a flat hand to gently compress the skin. Twist and push toward the lymph nodes (Figure 8–8). This stroke is very useful on the back of the torso and on the thighs, front and back. Repeat for a minute in one area before moving the hand to the next area. The "J" stroke can also be used toward the end of the massage, when the therapist is moving from the distal end of an extremity back toward the nodes. The most efficient way to use the "J" stroke is to move the hand closer toward the lymph nodes with each

(a)

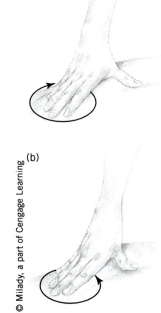

(b)

FIGURE 8–6 Stationary circle

© Milady, a part of Cengage Learning

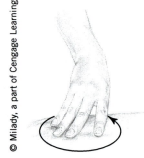

FIGURE 8–7 Pump

© Milady, a part of Cengage Learning

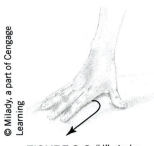

FIGURE 8–8 "J" stroke

© Milady, a part of Cengage Learning

repetition during the minute of massage, marching from the distal end of the extremity toward the nodes.

Effleurage

To perform effleurage, the therapist uses the flat palmar surface of the entire hand to first gently compress the skin, then sweep it toward the nodes (Figure 8–9). Repeat with one or both hands until there is a palpable change in the tissue. This stroke mechanically moves fluid, sweeping it through the lymphatics, but, because it only stretches the lymphatics in one direction, it is not as effective as movements that stretch the skin in a semicircle. It is, however, a useful stroke for self-massage.

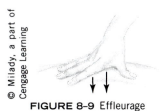

© Milady, a part of Cengage Learning

FIGURE 8-9 Effleurage

To save time, use two hands together to cover larger areas. Even though using two hands together saves time, the movements must still adhere to basic LDM principles: gentle, slow, rhythmic, repetitive strokes that move the skin.

It helps to visualize the movement of lymph during massage. Imagine hundreds of small streams converging to form a river that flows to the sea. LDM removes tiny blockages in the streams so that the fluid can flow freely toward its destination. Imagine that the work is smoothing the streambeds, coaxing rocks and other debris out of the way, and straightening the twists and bends to make the stream flow more easily.

Although therapists' hands do the work, it is important for the therapists to keep their body weight centered over the feet and to move from the body center. Therapists should move their bodies with the massage strokes. This slows the work and makes the pace more even. The client feels more grounded. When therapists stand with most of their body weight on one foot, or if they lean and stretch, the clients can feel the difference in the massage work and will sense that it is not as effective.

When working for a long time on one area of the body, it is often better to sit in a chair rather than stand. The therapist should pull the chair very close to the massage table, and sit back in the chair with the weight centered on the buttocks and the spine supported with the back of the chair. Therapists can still move their bodies with the massage strokes, moving from the hips. Keep both feet planted on the floor.

Pay close attention to subtle changes that occur in the tissue temperature, texture, and elasticity. As the work progresses, the skin should feel warmer, softer, looser, and more liquid. Skin that had been puffy or distended will begin to wrinkle slightly as the lymph fluid is drained from the area. Pay attention to the client's experience of the massage. Clients report such experiences as prickling sensations along the lymph pathways, heaviness, warmth, the need to urinate, and respiratory congestion during and after LDM.

LDM requires discipline and concentration. Before beginning the massage, the therapist should take a few moments to center and focus on the work to be done. The ability to focus on the work despite distractions is vital to success. Therapists who are distracted or daydream while giving massage will miss important, subtle changes in the tissue. With practice, and with discipline, therapists learn to sense the movement of lymph through tissues. Palpation skills become refined, and therapists move to new skill levels. This high level of sensitivity is worth the effort it takes to remain focused while doing repetitive work.

At the beginning of the massage, the massage therapist or esthetician should take a few moments to perform the following steps:

1. Check personal posture. The massage is more effective and feels better to clients when therapists have their weight centered on both feet, spine erect, head lifted, and chest expanded for easy breathing.

2. Concentrate on breathing slowly and regularly. Take a few slow breaths, inhaling through the nose and exhaling through the mouth with a slight pause at the end of each inhalation and exhalation.

3. Pay attention to the client's breathing. Is it regular or irregular, coming from the abdomen or chest, deep or shallow, fast or slow? When placing hands on the client's skin, take a moment to assess tissue condition. Is it cool or warm, pale or red, taut or flaccid? What is the extent and location of the edema, if any? Are there scars or other markings? Are there differences in the temperature of the skin in different areas? Are some areas more rigid than others?

4. During the massage, if distracted, repeat the preceding steps to regain focus. Pay attention to how the tissue changes during the session, and how the client responds. With practice and focus, it is possible to feel the movement of lymph through tissues. Because LDM is slow and repetitious, staying focused demands discipline on the part of the therapist. Discipline might be difficult at first, but it pays off in an increased ability to palpate subtle changes in the movement of tissue fluid.

REVIEW QUESTIONS

1. What is the purpose of moving the skin when applying LDM?

2. What is the optimal pressure for LDM?

3. Why is it important to repeat massage strokes when performing LDM and what is the recommended rate?

4. In what direction is the therapist trying to move the lymph when performing LDM?
   a. Toward the heart
   b. Toward the extremities
   c. Toward the lymph nodes

5. What is the basic pattern or order of movements in LDM?

6. What can happen if lymph nodes are not massaged before massaging an edematous area?

7. Why is slow, rhythmic repetition of strokes so important?
   a. To coordinate lymphatic contractions
   b. To stimulate a wave in lymph fluid
   c. To allow lymph to move at its own pace
   d. All of the above

8. What are watersheds?

9. From memory, draw a sketch of the pattern of lymph drainage to the trunk and

extremities. Include the watersheds and the location of lymph nodes.

10. Because of the watersheds, lymph can be directed around obstructions and drained toward the nodes on the unaffected side of the body.
    a. True
    b. False

11. Why is the well or unaffected side massaged first when working with obstructive edema?

12. What is the basic movement or stroke in LDM?

13. Why is the ability to focus and concentrate important in LDM? How can one increase the ability to concentrate?

14. What is the proper stance for the therapist when performing LDM? When seated?

The Lymph Drainage
Massage Session

This chapter covers communication, preparation for the massage session, the intake interview or consultation, beginning the massage, finishing the massage, recording client information, and setting up the next appointment.

COMMUNICATION

As every experienced therapist knows, there is more to massage than just bodywork. One of the most important factors in successful massage is communication. The therapist may have to coax the client to communicate not only factual information about health history and the client's background, but less clear-cut information about the client's assumptions and expectations regarding the massage and its outcome. The more information the therapist obtains from the client, the more successful the outcome of the massage.

Massage therapists must also clearly communicate their purpose for the massage, the kind of massage and its effects, what will happen during the session, the therapists' expectations about client participation in the session, and their expectations for the outcome of the massage. Also, therapists must communicate boundaries, policies, and procedures. This is time-consuming, so therapists should allow time for adequate communication, especially before and after the first LDM session.

The client may want some information about the therapist's background, education, and experience with LDM. A brochure or flyer with this information is useful. Therapists should also ask clients why they are having LDM, and what they expect the massage to achieve. Spend time educating the client, as there are many misconceptions about the purpose and effect of LDM.

Intake forms can save time and cover a lot of ground, so it is a good plan to have each new client fill one out. Allow clients to tell as much as they want about their health. People with chronic health problems may need to talk, and the information they provide is invaluable. When using intake forms, specifically ask about contraindications, and ask if there is any information the client thinks the therapist should know.

Explain procedures such as where the client will undress, where to hang clothes, where the massage will take place, and how to get on the massage table. Give the client control of the session: explain that the client has the right to ask questions, request changes, and give feedback to the therapist if he or she is hot, cold, uncomfortable, thirsty, or needs to use the bathroom.

Explain briefly how the massage will progress. Be sure to show the client where the lymph nodes are located, and explain why it is necessary to work in those areas. Because superficial lymph nodes are near private areas of the body, therapists should explain where they will put their hands and why. Doing so helps to develop trust between the client and therapist.

A wall chart that shows the locations of lymph nodes and the direction of lymph drainage helps to illustrate LDM. Do not assume that clients know this type of information. Most people lack accurate information about the lymphatic system.

INTAKE INTERVIEW OR CONSULTATION

Occasionally, a client will object to completing a health history. Explain that all kinds of massage, including LDM, cause physiological changes in the body, and that massage can adversely affect some pre-existing conditions. The therapist has a right and responsibility to request the information, and a client who is not willing to share the information is a poor risk for massage.

Clients may be concerned about confidentiality. Any business that collects health information is legally obliged to protect that information. Such information should be kept in a locked file accessible only to those who need to know the information. Therapists should never discuss a client's health information where it can be overheard by anyone other than the therapist and client. Client information should never be released to any third party without the client's written consent or a court order.

Clients' Records Should Include the Following Information:

Name, address, phone number

Physician's name and number

Emergency contact information

Reason for requesting LDM

Health history

—Diagnosis, where applicable

—Date of injury, when applicable

—Recent medical, chiropractic, or acupuncture treatment

—Medications and their purposes

Specifically ask about the contraindications. Remember that not all contraindications are absolute. Some conditions require the therapist to adapt the therapy to meet the client's needs. Specific questions for the intake session are described in Chapter Seven.

PREPARING FOR THE MASSAGE SESSION

Gather the necessary equipment and supplies. Set up the massage table with clean linen, a warm covering, a small neck roll for the client's neck, a half-bolster for the client's knees, and a full-round bolster for the client's ankles. Make sure the room has adequate ventilation, adequate indirect lighting, plenty of room to walk around the massage table, a rolling stool for the therapist, a small stool or chair for the client to use when dressing and undressing, a place to hang the client's clothes, and a place to store his/her personal items such as a purse, cell phone, or jewelry.

Music

Music is very useful during a massage session. Besides being a soothing sound that helps the client relax, the rhythm and pace of the music can help the therapist maintain the appropriate rhythm and pace of the massage movements. Appropriate music for lymph drainage massage is slow, soothing, approximately 60 beats per minute, and a little unpredictable so the client doesn't begin to sing along, or pay too much attention to the music and not enough to changes taking place in the body.

The Other Senses

Pay attention to the appearance of the massage room, which should be clean and uncluttered. Furnishings should be clean and not fussy. The same is true of the room's décor, which should be soothing rather than stimulating.

Clients experience lymph drainage massage on more than one level. While the therapist's skill and training are very important, therapists should also pay attention to details such as the smells in the room, background noises, and textures that will come into contact with the client's skin, such as those in the linens and bolsters.

Create a sense of sanctuary in the massage room, as this helps the client relax and develops trust. The client should feel safe in the therapist's hands. Trust develops when the therapist communicates clearly and shows a willingness to listen. It also helps when the therapist puts the client in control of the session, so that the client feels free to ask questions and express his or her needs. Clients are also reassured when a therapist clearly exhibits professionalism in communication, appearance and procedures.

BEFORE BEGINNING THE SESSION

At the beginning of the massage, the massage therapist or esthetician should take a few moments to perform the following steps:

1. Wash hands thoroughly.
2. Check personal posture. The massage is more effective and feels better to the client when the therapist has his/her weight centered on both feet, with spine erect, head lifted, and chest expanded for easy breathing.
3. Concentrate on breathing slowly and regularly. Take a few slow breaths, inhaling through the nose and exhaling through the mouth with a slight pause at the end of each inhalation and exhalation.
4. Pay attention to the client's breathing. Does it come from the abdomen or chest, is it regular or irregular, deep or shallow, fast or slow? When placing hands on the client's skin, take a moment to assess the tissue condition. Is it cool or warm, pale or flushed, taut or flaccid? What is the extent and location of the edema, if any? Are there scars or other markings? Are there differences in the temperature of the skin in different areas? Are some areas more rigid than others?
5. During the massage, if distracted, repeat preceding steps to regain focus. Pay attention to how the tissue changes during the session and how the client responds. With practice and focus, it is possible

to feel the movement of lymph through tissues. Because LDM is slow and repetitious, staying focused demands discipline on the part of the therapist. Discipline might be difficult at first, but it pays off in the increased ability to palpate subtle changes in the movement of tissue fluid.

BEGINNING THE SESSION

The massage begins with touch. Lay your hands on your client and let them rest there for a little while. Assess the state of the client's skin and underlying tissue—flexibility, tone, temperature, moisture, scar tissue, markings. Look for symmetry or asymmetry, palpate the tissue, and assess the amount of edema, fatty tissue, scar tissue, and fibrosis.

After the first few minutes of the session, when the client is visibly relaxing and demonstrating trust, encourage the client to rest quietly for a while. Some clients enjoy chatting with the therapist, but the therapist should remain focused on subtle changes in the tissue that indicate lymph movement, which is difficult if the therapist is also trying to carry on a conversation with the client about nonessentials.

Let the client know it is alright to ask questions about the work and to discuss anything else significant that may have been omitted from the intake interview, but subtly discourage chatter. Also, remind the client that it is alright to move the head, arms, or legs to be more comfortable and that it is alright to sigh, moan, snore, or make any other noise while relaxing.

Finish the session with gradually firmer pressure to signify the end of the massage, and the change from lymph work to a normal level of alertness. This should not be deep massage or heavy pressure, just a change in pressure and rhythm that signals the end of the massage. Use percussion or other stimulating techniques to ensure the client is awake enough to drive safely. Offer cold water to drink. Ask a few questions to make sure the client is fully aware of his/her surroundings.

If the client has been lying still for a half hour or more, it is helpful to stretch the client's lower back to prevent a cramp on arising. Ask the client to turn onto one side and to pull the knees to the chest for a few minutes, or ask the client to turn over and then massage the lower back. Help the client sit and then stand. Allowing the client to sit on the massage table with the feet dangling for a few minutes will raise the client's blood pressure, preventing fainting. Make sure the client is oriented to time and place and is not dizzy. Instruct the client in follow-up (e.g., exercises, other sessions, referrals to other practitioners). Be sure to offer a drink of water after the massage.

RECORDING CLIENT INFORMATION

After the session, record any additional information the client revealed about health history, the therapist's observations about the outcome of the massage, anything the client said about the effects of the massage, and any recommendations made by the therapist.

Client records serve several purposes. A good intake form can help gather information about the client's health history and activity level, give the therapist guidelines for discussing the client's massage expectations, and suggest areas of concern so that the therapist can ask more questions and make better, more informed decisions. Also, a good intake form documents that the therapist observed the contraindications and referred the client to medical practitioners when appropriate.

After the session, therapists should record each service or massage given to a client. Record observations, the client's report, the service/massage given to the client, and the outcomes and recommendations made to the client.

Occasionally, therapists are employed in facilities that do not use intake forms, such as spas and resorts. In these cases, therapists should discuss using intake forms with facility directors. When employers are unwilling to use intake forms, the therapist is responsible for asking each client for health information. Not doing so is malpractice.

Record changes in the client's health since the previous session. Record the client's report of the outcome of the previous session. Record the therapist's findings (location of swelling, pain, tightness, limited movement, skin condition). Record the outcome of the current session, and any recommendations made to the client or any referrals. Also, the therapist should include in the notes a record of any plans made with the client for the next session, such as the specific areas to be worked on, goals for the next massage, and any important reminders, such as a necessary follow-up with the client via phone call.

ACTIVITIES

1. Create a brochure describing the services you offer, such as LDM, and your training and background that qualify you to do the work. The brochure should serve two purposes: to disclose your qualifications and market your services.

2. If you work in a spa or other setting where intake forms are not used, set up a meeting with your director to discuss the need to inform clients of contraindications. Suggest having a copy of a pathology book for massage therapists at the front desk. Create a brochure that explains the most important contraindications for massage, and **encourages** clients **to** discuss their health history with their therapist.

Face and Neck Treatment Sequence

The head and neck are rich with lymph nodes, because disease-causing organisms can easily enter the body via the mouth, nose, and eyes. Lymph drainage massage stimulates the circulation of lymph and lymphocytes through the facial and cervical lymph nodes, which protect against those disease-causing organisms. LDM also removes excess fluid from the skin, preventing stagnation.

INDICATIONS AND CONTRAINDICATIONS

LDM to the face and neck very effectively reduces bruising and swelling following injury or surgery, including dental and cosmetic surgery. Because blood clots are a concern after surgery, LDM should not be offered until the client is released by the physician and requires no follow-up visits. Some physicians recommend LDM during healing. In that case, LDM should be performed according to the physician's instructions.

A physician should examine head and neck injuries to rule out serious conditions before massage is permissible. Open wounds, incisions, scratches, and abrasions should be allowed to heal before massage is offered.

Facial edema can be due to allergies, hormones, medication, fatigue, illness, infection, injury, excess salt in the diet, weeping, and so on. Because some of these conditions are contraindications, it is important to know the reason for the edema before proceeding. If the client is unsure and the edema persists, a medical examination may be in order before offering LDM. Once a proper diagnosis has been obtained and contraindications are ruled out, LDM may be used to reduce facial swelling.

Because lymph drainage massage stimulates the circulation of white blood cells, it helps to stimulate a sluggish immune system. It helps clients who frequently have minor illnesses. In fact, Dr. Vodder originally developed lymph drainage massage for this very purpose.

Similarly, LDM benefits clients with low energy. Low energy can result from stress, overwork, illness, or depression, any of which can depress the immune system. Stimulating immune circulation will help a fatigued client resist illness. In contrast, clients with high energy levels who overwork and overexercise are prone to illness and injuries because they do not rest. LDM is

Contraindications

- Thyroid disease
- Infection
- Acute inflammation
- Heart, liver or kidney failure
- Thrombosis, phlebitis
- Acute asthma
- Major surgery under general anesthesia
- Major injuries

© Milday, a part of Cengage Learning

deeply relaxing and may be used to help speed healing, as well as give overworked clients some rest.

Sometimes, clients who are fatigued believe they need deep massage work to feel better. Deep massage, or very firm pressure, can be exhausting and may require a few days of recovery time. Deep-tissue massage has its place, but it is inappropriate for clients who complain of fatigue. It may take some time to teach the client that deep work can be draining, and that subtle work is highly effective and will increase his or her energy level.

Although LDM is focused on superficial tissues, the muscles underneath also respond to the light, skillfully directed touch. Pain due to muscle tension will reduce or disappear. For instance, LDM can help relax the muscles that cause muscle-tension headaches. When facial muscles relax, the facial expression softens and relaxes, which contributes to a more youthful and healthy look.

LDM carries toxins (microscopic organisms, foreign particles, and the by-products of cellular energy combustion) away from the skin and allows increased nutrition to flow into the skin, improving its condition. Regular LDM changes the complexion, causing the skin to glow with increased health. If, however, the skin is infected, or if there is acne that is red and inflamed, it is better to wait until the infection has cleared before proceeding with any kind of facial massage.

Inflammation from injuries like whiplash causes edema because blood flow to the area increases, bringing a cleanup crew of cells to remove damaged cells and rebuild tissue. This can temporarily overload the local lymphatics. Also, muscles become rigid after an injury to protect the injured area from moving, making it more difficult for fluid to move out of the area. LDM stimulates lymph circulation, removing excess fluid from the area and helping the injury to heal faster. It also relaxes muscles, making them more flexible and improving the range of motion.

If there is a serious injury, massage is contraindicated until the injury has been examined to rule out fracture, torn ligaments, and so on. Once the injury has been examined by a physician and the acute symptoms have subsided, LDM is indicated to reduce swelling and speed healing. Once the injury has healed to the point that scar tissue has been deposited, LDM can be combined with connective tissue massage, such as deep-tissue massage or myofascial release. It helps reduce edema, it makes scar tissue softer and more flexible, and it helps contracted muscles relax.

Symptoms like stiffness, pain, limited movement, and muscle-tension headaches resulting from whiplash injuries can remain for years after the original injury. LDM and connective-tissue massage can improve matters even years after injury.

SWOLLEN LYMPH NODES

Chronically swollen lymph nodes can result from repeated infections and illnesses. Lymph nodes are considered to be abnormal if they are larger than one centimeter in diameter. It is important to have enlarged lymph nodes examined to rule out more serious conditions. If examination by a physician rules out any serious disease process, and no infection is present, regular LDM can help to reduce the size of the nodes and improve lymph circulation in the area. In this case, it is a good idea to teach the client to perform self-massage daily. Daily massage produces results faster.

LOCATING LYMPH NODES ON THE FACE AND NECK

The surface of the neck is divided into triangles to facilitate locating structures in the neck. (Figure 10–1) There are two large triangles—the anterior triangle and the posterior triangle. The anterior triangle is bordered by the sternocleido-mastoid muscle, the mandible, and the anterior midline. The posterior triangle is bordered by the sternocleidomastoid muscle, the clavicle and the trapezius muscle. Each of these large triangles is subdivided further by the digastric muscle and the omohyoid muscle.

The anterior triangle is divided into four smaller triangles by the anterior and posterior bellies of the digastric muscle, and the superior belly of the omohyoid muscle.

The submental triangle, under the chin, contains the submental lymph nodes and is located between the mandible, anterior belly of the digastric muscle, and the midline of the neck.

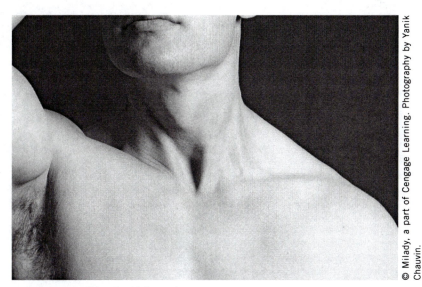

FIGURE 10-1 Triangles of the neck

The submandibular triangle, under the jaw, contains the submandibular lymph nodes and is located between the mandible, and the anterior and posterior bellies of the digastric muscle.

The carotid triangle contains important vessels of the neck, including the carotid artery, the internal jugular vein, the vagus nerve and the internal and external laryngeal nerves. It is bordered by the posterior belly of the digastric muscle, the superior belly of the omohyoid muscle and the sternocleidomastoid muscle.

The muscular triangle is bordered by the sternocleidomastoid muscle, the superior belly of the omohyoid muscle and the anterior midline of the neck. It contains important structures including the visceral column—a collective consisting of the thyroid, pharynx, larynx, trachea and esophagus.

The posterior triangle of the neck (sternocleidomastoid, clavicle and trapezius) is divided into the occipital triangle and the supraclavicular triangle by the inferior belly of the omohyoid muscle. The supraclavicular triangle contains the supraclavicular lymph nodes, and the occipital triangle contains the accessory lymph nodes.

Lymph nodes are located in the supraclavicular fossa, the neck, around the bottom of the head inferior to the base of occiput and the mandible, and in the face. (Figure 10–2)

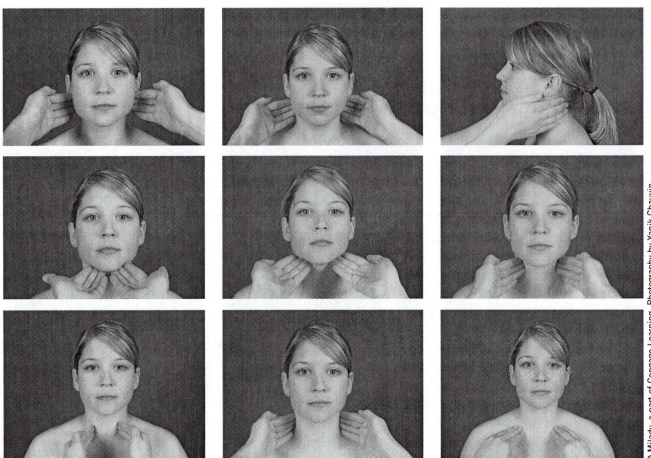

FIGURE 10–2 Lymph nodes of the head and neck

© Milady, a part of Cengage Learning. Photography by Yanik Chauvin.

TABLE 10–1

STRUCTURE	LOCATION	AFFERENTS FROM	EFFERENTS TO	REGIONS DRAINED
Right lymphatic duct[1]	Anterior to the anterior scalene, right side, looping above clavicle	Formed by the union of the right jugular trunk, right subclavian trunk, and right bronchomediastinal trunk	Junction of the right subclavian vein and right internal jugular vein	Right half of the head and neck; right upper limb; right side of the chest
Thoracic duct	Anterior to the anterior scalene, left side, looping above the clavicle	Formed by the union of the lumbar lymph trunks, sometimes dilated to form a cisterna chyli	Junction of the left subclavian vein And the left internal jugular vein	All of the body and limbs below the respiratory diaphragm; the left side of the chest, left upper limb and the left side of the head and neck
Jugular trunk	Carotid sheath in root of neck	Deep cervical nodes	Left: thoracic duct, right: right lymphatic duct, or junction of right subclavian and right internal jugular vein	Lymphatic vessels of the head and neck
Supraclavicular nodes (part of inferior deep cervical nodes)	In and around carotid sheath below level of omohyoid	Superior deep cervical nodes, transverse cervical nodes, accessory nodes	Efferents join to form the jugular lymphatic trunk	Head and neck

(Continued)

STRUCTURE	LOCATION	AFFERENTS FROM	EFFERENTS TO	REGIONS DRAINED
Superior deep cervical nodes[2]	In and around carotid sheath posterior and lateral to the internal jugular vein	Lymphatic vessels and numerous node groups from the head and neck	Inferior deep cervical nodes	Head and neck
Inferior deep cervical nodes	Around the internal jugular vein, inferior to the crossing of the omohyoid muscle	Superior deep cervical nodes	Jugular trunk	Head and neck
Jugulodigastric node	Anterolateral to internal jugular vein where it is crossed by posterior belly of the digastric	Part of the superior deep cervical nodes	Inferior deep cervical nodes	Oral cavity, tongue, palatine tonsil
Juguloomohyoid node	Lateral to internal jugular vein where it is crossed by superior belly of omohyoid	Superior deep cervical nodes	Inferior deep cervical nodes	Submental region and tip of tongue
Transverse cervical nodes	Along the course of the transverse cervical blood vessels	Accessory chain of nodes, sometimes the apical axillary nodes	Jugular lymphatic trunk, right lymphatic duct or thoracic duct, jugular or subclavian vein	Lateral part of the neck, anterior thoracic wall, mammary gland
Superficial cervical nodes[3]	In superficial fascia and along superficial vessels of the neck	Lymphatic vessels from superficial structures in head and neck	Varies by group; ultimate destination is the jugular trunk	Head and neck
Occipital nodes	Superior nuchal line, over the insertion of the semispinalis capitis muscle, between insertion of SCM and occipital attachment of trapezius	Posterior scalp	Accessory nodes	Occipital part of the scalp and the superior neck
Retroauricular nodes	Posterior to the ear, at the insertion of the SCM	Lymphatic vessels from the ear and side of the head	Superior deep cervical nodes	Scalp overlying the posterior temporoparietal region; posterior ear
Submental nodes	Under the mandible on the mylohyoid muscle	Lymphatic vessels from the lower face and chin	Submandibular nodes, juguloomohyoid node	Tip of the tongue, lower lip, floor of the mouth, chin, lower gums
Submandibular nodes	Inferior and medial to the mandible	Submental nodes; facial nodes; lymphatic vessels from the submandibular and sublingual regions	Superior deep cervical nodes; juguloomohyoid node	Anterior part of tongue, lower lip, floor of the mouth, nose, cheeks, chin, gums and lower incisor teeth, lower surface of palate
Anterior jugular nodes	Along the anterior jugular vein	Lymphatic vessels of the anterior inferior part of the neck	Inferior deep cervical nodes	Skin and muscle of the anterior infrahyoid region of the neck
External jugular nodes	Along the external jugular vein	Lymphatic vessels from the side of the head	Superior deep cervical nodes	Inferior part of the ear and the parotid region
Deep parotid nodes	On the lateral side of the pharyngeal wall, deep to the parotid gland	Lymphatic vessels from the ear	Superior deep cervical nodes	External opening to the ear, auditory tube, middle ear

STRUCTURE	LOCATION	AFFERENTS FROM	EFFERENTS TO	REGIONS DRAINED
Accessory nodes	Posterior triangle of the neck, arranged along the accessory nerve	Occipital nodes, retroauricular nodes	Transverse cervical chain of nodes	Occipital region and posterior scalp, posterior neck and supraspinatus region
Parotid nodes, superficial	Superficial to the parotid salivary gland over the masseter muscle	Anterior auricular nodes	Superior deep cervical nodes	Skin of the anterior ear and its external opening, temporal and frontal area, eyelids, lacrimal gland, cheek and nose, posterior and floor of nasal cavities
Anterior auricular nodes	Anterior to the tragus of the ear, inferior to the zygomatic arch	Lymphatic vessels from the side of the head	Superior parotid nodes; superior deep cervical nodes	Anterior part of the temporoparietal region of the scalp; anterior surface of the ear and external opening to the ear
Infraorbital nodes	Infraorbital region from the nasolabial groove to the zygomatic arch	Lymphatic vessels from the face	Submandibular nodes	Eyelids, nose, cheek
Buccal nodes	Superior to the buccinators muscle, near the corner of the lips	Lymphatic vessels from the face	Deep cervical nodes	Cheek
Juxtavisceral nodes[4]	Adjacent to the esophagus, larynx, trachea and thyroid gland	Cervical viscera	Superior deep cervical nodes, inferior deep cervical nodes	Esophagus, larynx, trachea and thyroid gland
Tonsil, lingual	Superior surface of the root of the tongue	Tongue	Superior deep cervical nodes	Protect against pathogens that are inhaled or swallowed
Tonsil, palatine[5]	Lateral wall of the oropharynx between the palatoglossal and palatopharyngeal arches	Lymphatic vessels of the posterior tongue and palatoglossal/palatopharyngeal arch region	Superior deep cervical nodes, especially the jugulodigastric node	Protect against pathogens that are inhaled or swallowed
Tonsil, pharyngeal	Near the posterior openings of the nasal cavity	Lymphatic vessels of the wall of the pharynx	Superior deep cervical nodes	Protect against pathogens that are inhaled or swallowed
Tonsil, tubal	At the pharyngeal opening of the auditory tube[6]	Lymphatic vessels of the auditory tube	Superior deep cervical nodes	Protect the entrance to the nasopharynx

[1]The right lymphatic duct doesn't always exist. Instead, the three trunks that form right lymphatic duct sometimes connect directly to the venous system.

[2]Superior and inferior subdivisions of deep cervical nodes are delineated by the crossing of the omohyoid muscle.

[3]Several groups are designated by location: occipital, retroauricular, anterior auricular, submental, submandibular, external jugular, anterior jugular.

[4]Includes: infrahyoid, prelaryngeal, pretracheal and paratracheal nodes.

[5]Palatine, lingual and pharyngeal tonsils form the tonsillar ring (of Waldeyer).

[6]Tube that connects the ear to the nasal cavity.

Source: MedCharts Anatomy by Gest, Thomas R. and Schlesinger, Jaye, MedCharts Anatomy, ILOC, Inc., New York. 1995. Feltman, Barbara; Petterborg, Larry. "Lymph flow of the digestive tract." Rehabilitation Oncology. 2002 University of Arkansas for Medical Sciences: Table of Lymphatics of the Abdomenhttp://anatomy.uams.edu/anatomyhtml/lymph_abdomen.html, accessed February, 2010.

Massage should begin with the supraclavicular lymph nodes and then continue with the cervical lymph nodes along the sternocleidomastoid muscle from the origin to the insertion, including the belly of the muscle, and the medial and lateral borders of the muscle.

Next, the lymph nodes in a ring around the bottom of the head should be massaged, including the submental, submandibular, postauricular and occipital nodes.

Finally the lymph nodes of the face should be massaged, beginning with the preauricular and parotid nodes, and following with the facial nodes, from the infraorbital region, just below the eyes, down past the corner of the mouth.

After draining the tissues of the head and neck, the lymph nodes should be massaged again, in reverse order, ending at the supraclavicular nodes.

OBSERVING AND PALPATING LYMPH NODES ON THE FACE AND NECK

Before proceeding, and while the client is seated and facing the therapist, look carefully at the client's face and neck. Look for asymmetry and any swelling or signs of inflammation in front of or behind the ears, under the eyes, along the jawline, in the neck, and in the supraclavicular triangle. In a healthy person, the lymph nodes should not be visibly swollen or inflamed. (Figure 10–3) When

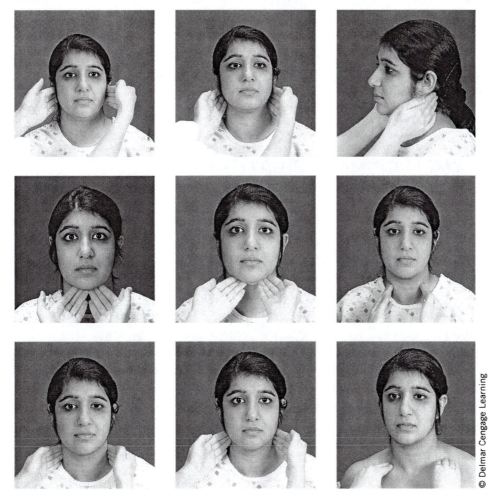

© Delmar Cengage Learning

FIGURE 10–3 Palpation of cervical and facial lymph nodes

swelling or inflammation is present, discuss the condition with the client before proceeding. If the client does not know the reason for the swelling or inflammation and has never had it examined, do *not* proceed with the massage until a physician has ruled out serious health conditions. Swollen lymph nodes indicate infection, which is a contraindication for massage. For instance, swollen lymph nodes under the jawline can indicate a dental infection, swollen tonsils can indicate a sinus infection, and swollen nodes near the ear can indicate an ear infection. Swollen nodes can also indicate a more serious health problem, such as cancer, so the client should definitely be examined by a physician.

Chronically enlarged lymph nodes may be due to a serious underlying health problem, such as sinusitis or tonsillitis, or other chronic infections. Lymph nodes can also be scarred by repeated infections and remain enlarged after the infection has disappeared.

After observing the lymph nodes, the next step is to palpate the lymph nodes. When the client is lying supine on the massage table, palpate the lymph nodes of the neck and face. Using medium to light pressure, massage in small circles over the areas where the lymph nodes are located, attempting to locate small, pea-sized masses that can be moved. Palpate the tissues behind and in front of the ears (post- and preauricular lymph nodes), under the jawline from the chin (submental lymph nodes) to the angle of the jaw (submandibular lymph nodes), and inferior to the occipital ridge along the hairline. Palpate along the sternocleidomastoid muscle and in the tissues that are medial and lateral to the SCM. Palpate between the SCM and the trapezius muscle (posterior cervical chain and accessory lymph nodes), and in the supraclavicular triangle.

At the same time, observe and palpate any areas of edema and any scar tissue. Edema indicates blocked or overloaded lymph circulation, and scar tissue inhibits the circulation of lymph.

LYMPH DRAINAGE PATHWAYS ON THE FACE AND NECK

Lymphatic vessels of the head and neck drain inferiorly, from the scalp to the jugular trunks which connect to the jugular or subclavian veins via the thoracic duct and the right lymphatic duct. (Figure 10–4)

The posterior scalp drains inferiorly toward the occipital and post-auricular lymph nodes. The parietal and temporal regions of the scalp drain toward the closest nodes, so some lymph vessels on the top of the head drain to the occipital and post-auricular lymph nodes, and some to the preauricular nodes and then to the submandibular nodes. On the face, the frontal and temporal regions drain toward the preauricular lymph nodes. The ear and tissues around and inside the ear drain both to the preauricular and postauricular lymph nodes. The front of the face drains from the eyes, nose and mouth inferiorly to the submandibular and submental lymph nodes. The sides of the face drain toward the preauricular lymph nodes, and then the submandibular lymph nodes.

After passing through all these nodes, lymph from the head enters the cervical chains. The superficial cervical chain drains the skin of the head and neck, and the deep chain drains the tongue, the inside of the mouth, the thyroid and

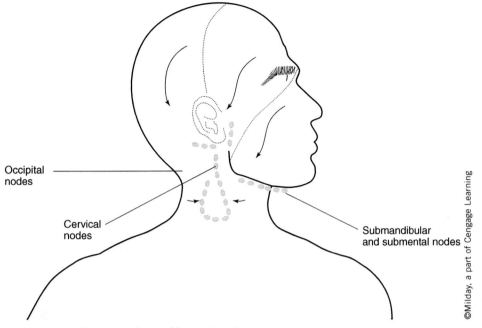

Occipital
nodes

Cervical
nodes

Submandibular
and submental nodes

FIGURE 10-4 Drainage patterns of face and neck

deeper tissues of the neck. From the cervical lymph nodes, fluid drains into the jugular trunks and thence to the jugular or subclavian vein via the thoracic duct or the right lymphatic duct.

Procedure for lymph drainage massage of head and neck LDM is performed on both sides of the neck and face at the same time, although the directions only mention one side. Use both hands and work both sides at the same time. Unless indicated otherwise, use stationary circles. Repeat stationary circles until the tissue feels softer, it is easier to palpate deeper structures, and the skin stretches in a larger circle. Massage for at least a minute, up to three minutes if necessary. Complete seven to ten repetitions per minute.

It is more important to understand the lymph drainage patterns of the head and neck than to memorize a one-size-fits-all massage sequence. It is also important to develop good palpation skills, so as to be able to sense the movement of lymph fluid through the tissues during massage. Then the therapist or esthetician can tailor each massage session to the needs of the individual client, and spend more time on the areas that need the most work.

MASSAGE OUTLINE

1. Wash hands thoroughly.
2. Gather equipment and supplies. Adjust the height of the table. Use bolsters, if needed, for the client's legs. Place a small bolster beneath the client's knees, and a slightly larger bolster under the client's ankles. If the room is cool, cover the client.
3. Sit or stand at the client's head. Carefully drape a warm, moist towel over the client's face, leaving room for the client to breathe. Allow the towel to cool to room temperature. As the towel cools, massage gently

through the towel to relax the tissues. Before removing the towel, use it to gently wipe the face.

4. Optionally, apply warm lotion to the skin with smooth strokes, covering the face and the front and back of the neck. Lotion or cream isn't necessary, but it is recommended because some clients may worry about the skin being stretched or irritated, and the lotion or moisturizer is very soothing. Avoid applying so much lotion or cream that it becomes difficult to move the skin without sliding over it.

Massaging the Neck

Massage each set of lymph nodes for at least a minute, until the tissue seems warmer, more flexible and can be moved around in larger circles.

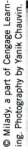

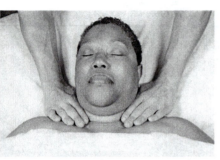

FIGURE 10–5 Supraclavicular lymph nodes

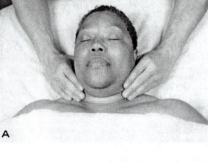

A

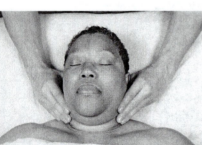

B

FIGURE 10–6 A & B Cervical chains

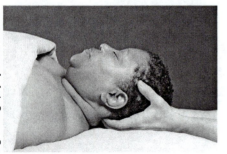

FIGURE 10–7 Suboccipital lymph nodes

Massage the back of the neck between the hairline and the spine of the scapula, using flat fingers to move the skin in gentle circles.

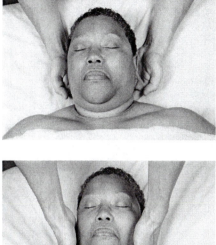

Massage the sides of the neck between the ear and the collar.

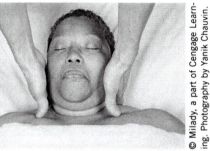

Massage the front of the neck over the visceral column, which contains the esophagus, trachea and thyroid.

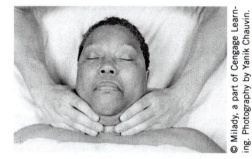

Massage the area of the submandibular and submental triangles.

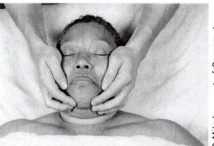

Gently effleurage the back of the neck from the cervical spine forward to the sternocleidomastoid muscles.

Gently effleurage the front of the neck from the midline laterally toward the sternocleidomastoid muscles.

Massaging the Head

Continue massaging the ring of lymph nodes around the bottom of the head that drain the vessels from the face and scalp.

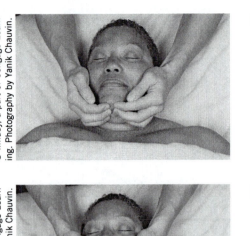

Start with the submental lymph nodes.

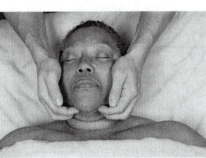

Next, massage the submandibular lymph nodes.

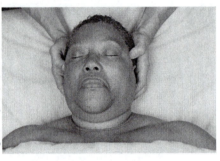

Massage the postauricular lymph nodes.

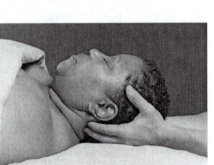

Finish with the occipital lymph nodes.

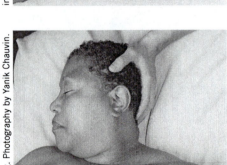

Massage the posterior scalp, turning the head as necessary to work all areas.

Massage the top of the head.

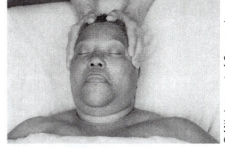

Massage the frontal region between the eyebrows and the anterior hairline moving lymph laterally toward the pre-auricular nodes.

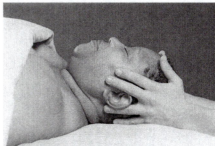

Massage the temporal region.

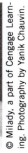

Massage in front of and behind the ears (fork.)

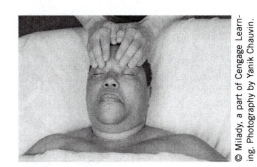

Massage the eyebrows and upper lids.

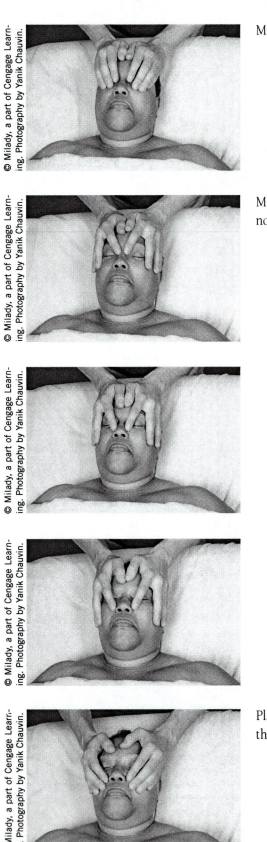

Massage the infraorbital area gently with the fingertips.

Massage the root of the nose, then the bridge, and then the wings of the nose.

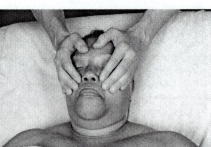

Place fingertips in the nasolabial groove, and massage the area between the eyes and lips with flat fingers.

Massage the cheeks over the teeth.

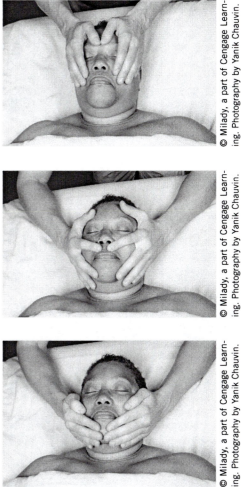

Massage above and below the lips.

Massage the chin.

Massage the lymph nodes again, in reverse order: infraorbital, pre-auricular and superficial parotid, then the lymph nodes around the bottom of the head: submental, submandibular, post-auricular and occipital nodes. Then massage the accessory and cervical lymph nodes, and the supraclavicular lymph nodes.

Finish the massage with very light effleurage or delicate tapotement with fingertips over the face and neck.

Lymph drainage massage of the head and neck can be offered with a body wrap, but the therapist must be sure the client does not become dehydrated. Offer the client water before the session begins, and have a glass of water with a flexible straw available during the session.

If the purpose of the treatment is to enhance the immune system during or before flu season, urge the client to have three to seven sessions in one week. While this frequency of sessions is very beneficial, it is intense, and mind-body reactions or healing crises are possible. Be sure to read the material on those subjects later in this text. Students who are practicing this massage sequence may find it tedious to keep counting the seconds and numbers of circles. However, the results are worth the effort. Success depends on the rhythm and rate of repetitions, and the best way to ensure perfect rhythm, speed and rate of repetitions is to count the seconds and number of circles. Use music with 60 beats per minute or a clock with an unobtrusive ticking sound. This is a very delightful massage experience for the client. Not only does it stimulate lymph circulation, it is deeply relaxing. With appropriate music, soft lighting, subtle aromatherapy, and carefully selected emollient, as well as a skillful, directed touch, the client will experience the work on more than one level and can find the experience profound.

Lymph Drainage Massage of the Upper Extremities and Trunk

INDICATIONS

Edema of the upper extremities can arise from injury, repetitive motion strain, scar tissue, and more serious conditions, such as the scar tissue and obstruction that result from cancer surgery and radiation treatment. When edema due to obstruction becomes chronic, it is called lymphedema disease. Lymphedema disease progresses over time and, at the least, is uncomfortable and reduces quality of life, affecting daily activities. At the worst, lymphedema disease results in chronic serious infections. At this stage, it is painful and impacts seriously on the quality of life and makes daily activities difficult, if not impossible.

Lymphedema is a progressive disorder that cannot be cured, although it does respond well to LDM, bandaging, and exercise, often called comprehensive decongestive therapy. Ideally, clients with lymphedema would be referred by their physicians to therapists with advanced training in these areas. However, there are too few LDM therapists in the United States to treat the number of people with obstructive edema or lymphedema. Therapists should not be afraid to help any clients who come to them with edema. Therapists should review the contraindications with every client so as to avoid doing harm. If a client has lymphedema disease in the third or fourth stage (see the discussion on staging of lymphedema elsewhere in the text), any kind of massage should be given only under a physician's supervision.

Scar tissue responds slowly to massage, and takes repeated sessions to obtain visible results. Progress is faster if LDM is combined with connective tissue massage, such as skin rolling or cross-fiber friction.

Inflammation resulting from overuse, such as carpal tunnel syndrome, tennis elbow, or frozen shoulder, responds well to lymph drainage massage. LDM speeds healing, reduces inflammation, reduces pain, and improves circulation and flexibility. Generally, clients with these conditions also need deeper massage on the overworked muscles that are involved to stretch and relax these muscles, and possibly movement training to change or eliminate the movement causing the problem.

LDM is indicated for painful, swollen breasts due to the hormone fluctuations involved with the menstrual cycle, pregnancy, or birth control pills. It is important for women who wear constricting brassieres to perform self-massage on their breasts regularly. Lymph vessels are close to the surface of the skin, and tight bras that leave lines in the skin when removed are compressing the lymph vessels in the breast area, leading to sluggish or obstructed lymph flow. Over years, this can contribute to increased infections and other breast problems.

LOCATING AXILLARY AND BREAST LYMPH NODES

Lymph nodes of the upper quadrants and upper extremities include the axillary nodes (apical, central, pectoral, subscapular and lateral nodes), the infraclavicular and supraclavicular nodes, the cubital nodes and the internal mammary chain.

Most of the lymph fluid from the superficial tissues of the chest, breast, and upper extremities drains into the pectoral, subscapular, and lateral nodes, and

from those three groups into the central and apical axillary nodes. (Table 11–1)
From the central and apical axillary nodes, fluid travels to the infraclavicular
and supraclavicular nodes, and subclavian trunk. Some of the lymph from the

TABLE 11–1 Lymph Nodes In The Upper Trunk

STRUCTURE	LOCATION	AFFERENTS FROM	EFFERENTS TO	REGIONS DRAINED
Subclavian trunk	Along the course of the subclavian vein	Apical axillary nodes; infraclavicular nodes	Joins the jugular trunk on the right to form the right lymphatic duct; empties into the thoracic duct on the left	Upper arms, most of the mammary glands, the anterolateral chest wall
Supraclavicular nodes	Supraclavicular triangle	Accessory chain of nodes, sometimes the apical axillary nodes	Variable: jugular lymphatic trunk, right lymphatic trunk or thoracic duct	Lateral part of the neck, the anterior thoracic wall, mammary glands
Infraclavicular nodes	Along the cephalic vein in the deltopectoral groove	Lymphatic vessels from the superficial upper arm	Apical axillary nodes	Skin and the superficial fascia of the upper arms
Sternal nodes	Lateral border of the sternum, intercostal spaces 1 to 6	Anterior phrenic nodes, lymphatic vessels from the anterior thoracic wall	Trunks in the lower neck	Medial side of the mammary glands, anterior chest wall and muscles
Apical axillary nodes	Apex of the axilla	Lateral, central, subscapular and pectoral nodes, the lymph vessels of the mammary glands, and along the cephalic vein	Subclavian lymphatic trunk, deep cervical lymph nodes	Upper arms, most of the mammary glands, some of the anterolateral chest wall, the posterior thoracic wall and the scapular region
Central axillary nodes	In the center of the axilla, along the ribs	Lateral, pectoral and subscapular nodes; mammary glands and upper arms	Apical axillary nodes	Upper arms, mammary glands, the anterior and lateral chest wall, the posterior thoracic wall and scapular region
Lateral axillary nodes (brachial nodes)	In the axilla, along the humerus	Cubital nodes, lymphatic vessels of the arm	Central axillary nodes, apical axillary nodes	Upper arms
Subscapular axillary nodes (posterior axillary nodes)	In the axilla, anterior to the posterior wall of the axilla, which is formed by the teres major and latissimus dorsi muscles	Back of the neck, upper back, scapular muscles	Central axillary nodes	Back of the neck, upper back, scapular muscles
Pectoral axillary nodes (anterior axillary nodes)	In the axilla, posterior to the anterior axillary wall, which is formed by the pectoralis major muscle	Lymphatic vessels from the mammary glands and anterolateral thoracic wall	Central axillary nodes	Anterolateral thoracic wall and muscles, mammary glands
Cubital nodes (epitrochlear)	Medial end of the cubital fossa	Lymphatic vessels from the forearm, ulnar side	Lateral axillary nodes	Ulnar side of the forearm and hand

breast area drains into the sternal nodes, and then into the lymphatic trunks of the lower neck.

Axillary lymph nodes are easily located. With the client lying supine on the table, rotate the arm so the arm is abducted from the body, with the hand near the top of the head. If necessary, support the arm with a pillow so that the arm and shoulder are relaxed. Locate the central and apical axillary nodes by placing the fingers deep into the center of the axilla, and press the tissue gently against the thoracic wall. Massage in gentle circles to locate the nodes.

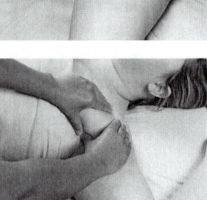

Locate the central and apical axillary nodes by placing the fingers deep into the center of the axilla, and press the tissue gently against the thoracic wall. Massage in gentle circles to locate the nodes.

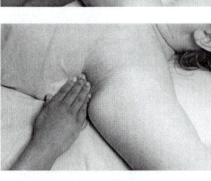

Locate the pectoral nodes between the lateral edge of the pectoralis major muscle (the anterior wall of the axilla) and the ribs. Press into the posterior side of the pectoralis major muscle.

Locate the subscapular nodes at the anterior edge of the latissimus dorsimuscle (the posterior wall of the axilla).

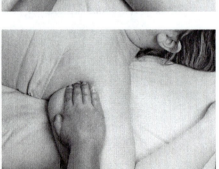

The brachial nodes are located on the inner aspect of the arm, near the axilla, along the humerus.

To locate the supraclavicular nodes, place the fingertips above the upper border of the clavicle, in the supraclavicular triangle.

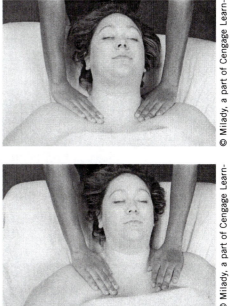

To locate the infraclavicular nodes, place the fingertips just below the lower border of the clavicle, in the deltopectoral groove.

The lymph nodes should not be painful to the touch, and they should be very small. Nodes that are enlarged and painful when palpated indicate infection, and the client should be referred to a physician. Likewise, enlarged nodes that are fixed, or immovable, may indicate a possibly serious health problem, and the client should be referred to a physician. Once the condition has been examined by a physician and serious health conditions have been ruled out, it is safe to proceed with the massage.

MASSAGE OF THE UPPER EXTREMITY AND TRUNK

With the client lying in a supine position, massage the lymph nodes first, beginning with the supraclavicular and infraclavicular nodes on both sides of the body at the same time. Then massage the axillary nodes on the unaffected side of the body. The purpose is to establish normal circulation and rhythm in the unaffected areas of the upper body, and make space so that blocked tissue fluid on the affected side of the body can be moved around obstructions to the lymphatic vessels on the unaffected side.

Massage the anterior proximal quadrant of the trunk on the unaffected side, around the breast tissue, moving lymph toward the axillary nodes. Begin proximal to the nodes and work toward the sternum and the lower margin of the ribs.

Repeat the massage of the axillary nodes and upper anterior trunk quadrant on the affected side of the body.

Massage the upper limb on the affected side, moving lymph toward the axillary nodes. Massage the proximal areas first (deltoid area, followed by biceps brachii and triceps brachii areas), and continue massaging distally to the ends of the fingers.

Massage the arm in reverse, from the fingers to the axilla again. Then ask the client to change to a prone position so that the posterior upper quadrant can be massaged. Begin near the axillary lymph nodes, massaging over the scapula and working outward, toward the midline and the lower margin of the ribs. Be sure to also massage the lateral aspect of the ribs.

Finish the massage by massaging the lymph nodes again in reverse order. Massage the cubital nodes, axillary nodes, infraclavicular, and then supraclavicular nodes.

DETAILED MASSAGE OUTLINE

Unless otherwise indicated, use stationary circles. Each circle should last 7 seconds and should be repeated for at least a minute, until the tissue becomes softer, warmer, and can be stretched in larger circles. Remember to compress the skin slightly with your fingers and stretch the skin around toward the lymph nodes in a semicircle, then reduce the pressure and ride the skin back toward the starting point.

Gather equipment and supplies. Help the client onto the table, and drape warmly. Begin with the client in the supine position.

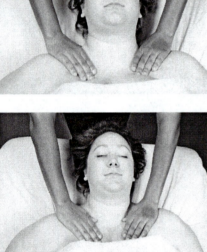

Standing at the client's head, massage the supraclavicular nodes bilaterally, using both hands, for at least a minute.

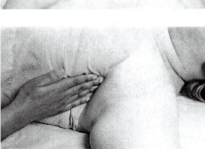

Massage the infraclavicular nodes bilaterally.

Standing at the client's unaffected side, massage the axillary nodes. Central and apical axillary nodes: Place the fingers at the apex of the axilla between the pectoralis major and the latissimus dorsi muscle, touching the thoracic wall. Massage using stationary circles for at least one minute.

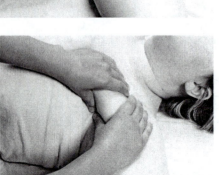

Anterior (pectoral) nodes: Place the fingertips beneath the pectoralis major muscle at the front wall of the axilla, and massage for at least one minute.

© Milady, a part of Cengage Learning. Photography by Yanik Chauvin.

Posterior (subscapular) nodes: Place the fingertips on the border of the latissimus dorsi muscle at the back wall of the axilla, and massage for at least one minute.

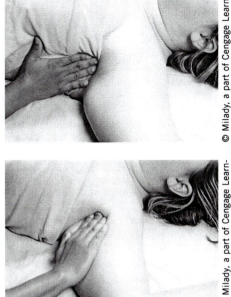

Lateral (brachial) nodes: With the client's arm raised above the head and supported on a pillow, if necessary, place the entire hand over the brachial nodes along the humerus, with the fingers touching the center of the axilla, and massage for at least one minute.

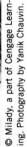

Massage the anterior trunk quadrant adjacent to the lymph nodes on the unaffected side. Begin proximal to the nodes and work toward the midline and the lower margin of the ribs around the breast tissue, moving lymph toward the axillary lymph nodes. At each step, massage for about one minute, using stationary circles. Count seven seconds percircle.

Place a flat hand over the shoulder joint between the deltoid muscle and breast. Massage for at least a minute, until the tissue is soft and flexible, and can be stretched in a larger circle than at the beginning.

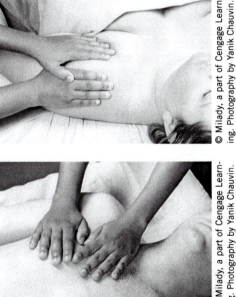

Massage the area of the pectoralis major. For a male client, simply place both flat hands to cover the upper half of the pectoralis major, and massage for at least one minute. Then, use both hands to cover the lower portion of the pectoralis major, below the nipple, and massage for one minute. Place one hand over the sternum and massage for one minute.

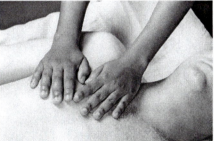

For a female client, place one hand along the lower margin of the clavicle, above the breast, and massage for at least one minute, moving fluid toward the axillary nodes.

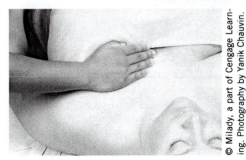

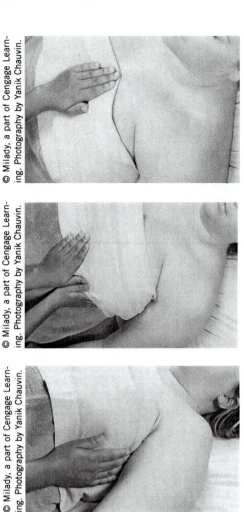

© Milady, a part of Cengage Learning. Photography by Yanik Chauvin.

Then place one hand over the sternum and massage for at least one minute, moving fluid superiorly toward the base of the neck.

© Milady, a part of Cengage Learning. Photography by Yanik Chauvin.

Place both hands below the breast and massage for at least one minute, moving fluid toward the axillary nodes.

© Milady, a part of Cengage Learning. Photography by Yanik Chauvin.

Place one hand on the lateral margin of the breast (ask the client to move the breast tissue out of the way) and massage for at least one minute, moving fluid toward the axillary nodes.

The female breast will definitely benefit from lymph drainage massage. However, in many places in the United States, it is illegal for massagetherapists to touch the female breast. This isn't true in every country. In any case, teaching clients to massage their own breasts at home is important. Before or after the session, explain and demonstrate selfmassage so that the client can do it herself at home.

Use one or two hands to massage the lower rib cage for at least one minute.

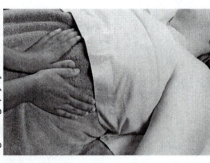

© Milady, a part of Cengage Learning. Photography by Yanik Chauvin.

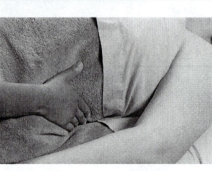

© Milady, a part of Cengage Learning. Photography by Yanik Chauvin.

Use one or two hands to cover the lateral wall of the thorax between the bottom of the ribs and the axilla, and massage for at least oneminute.

Repeat the massage to the axillary nodes and the anterior upper quadrant on the affected side of the body. Massage the upper limb on the affected side of the body. Massage from proximal to distal on the limb using stationary circles for at least one minute over each of the following areas:

Deltoid muscle area (cap of the shoulder)

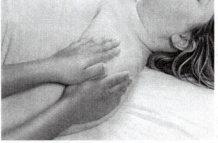
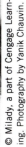

Front of the upper arm, over the biceps brachii muscle

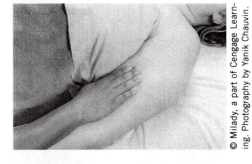

Front of the upper arm, on the tissue on both sides of the biceps brachii muscle

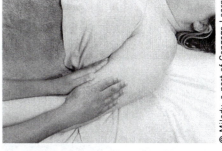
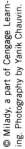

Medial and lateral ends of the elbow crease

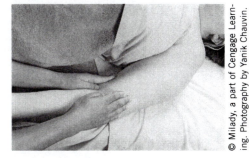

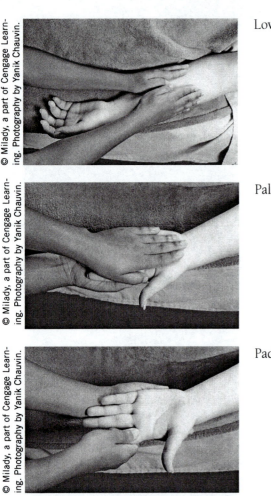

© Milady, a part of Cengage Learning. Photography by Yanik Chauvin.

Lower arm

Palm of the hand

Pads of the fingers and thumb

The dorsum of the hand

Reverse the previous steps and massage from the hand to the shoulder.Help the client turn over to a prone position. Massage the posteriortrunk quadrant, beginning close to the lymph nodes and working outward toward the midline and the lower margin of the ribs. Massage each of the following.

Shoulder joint

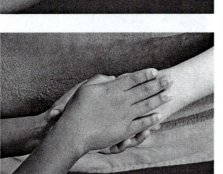

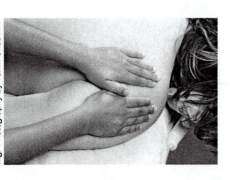

© Milady, a part of Cengage Learning. Photography by Yanik Chauvin.

Lateral edge of scapula

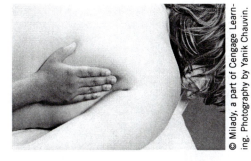

Scapula

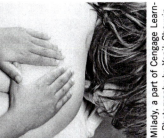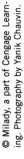

Back of the neck

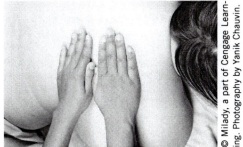

Upper trapezius

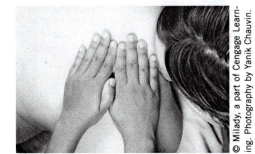

Middle trapezius

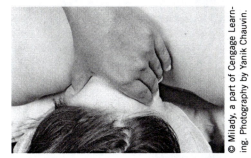

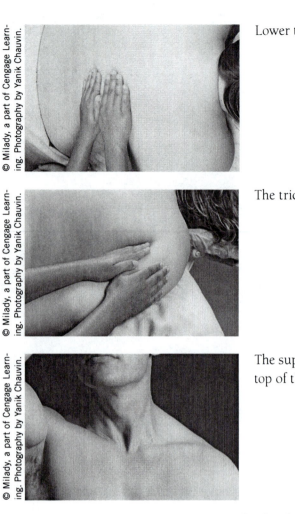

© Milady, a part of Cengage Learning. Photography by Yanik Chauvin.

Lower trapezius

The triceps muscle, using one or both hands

The supraclavicular triangle. Place a hand on the trapezius muscle at the top of the shoulder and curve the fingers under to reach the clavicle.

Help the client turn over again to a supine position. Massage over the axillary lymph nodes, then the infraclavicular and supraclavicular nodes again, to complete this quadrant.

Finish with gentle effleurage.

If you discover a lump in the tissue during the massage, or the client reports finding a lump, recommend that the client see a physician to identify it. Don't alarm the client, but also don't minimize the importance of seeing a doctor for examination.

Teach clients self-massage for the breast. See Chapter 16 for details.

Lymph Drainage Massage on the Lower Extremities and Trunk

INDICATIONS AND CONTRAINDICATIONS

Edema of the lower leg can be due to injury, repetitive-motion strain, scar tissue, or more serious conditions, such as the scar tissue and obstruction that result from cancer surgery. It can sometimes be caused simply by the position of the leg and foot; for example, when sitting for a long time without moving, tissue fluid pools in the lower leg. Edema of the lower limb can also be due to obstruction of the lymph nodes from the weight gain of pregnancy or obesity, or tight clothing such as socks or stockings. All these conditions respond to LDM.

Edema of the lower leg is an indication for LDM. LDM moves fluid out of the tissue spaces into the lymphatic vessels so that it can be returned to the bloodstream. LDM also improves the appearance and texture of the skin, which can become stiff, coarse, and reddened because of chronic edema.

However, edema of the lower leg is also a symptom of a variety of serious illnesses, such as congestive heart failure and kidney failure. Edema of the legs and hands should be referred to a physician to rule out serious underlying illnesses before proceeding, unless the cause of the edema is obvious, such as a long period of enforced sitting on a plane, for instance, or a known side effect of medication.

If a client has been sitting for a long time on a car ride or flight, a blood clot is possible. If the lower leg is red, hot, painful, and swollen, do not massage. If there is sharp pain, do not massage. In either case, refer to a physician to rule out a blood clot.

Before beginning to massage, look for varicose veins. If these are inflamed and painful, no massage should be given until the condition has been examined by a physician. If the veins are not painful and are not red, hot, and swollen, light massage such as that associated with LDM is safe. It is generally safe to massage over spider veins and small broken capillaries.

LDM helps speed healing of injuries by stimulating microcirculation, assisting in the removal of cellular debris from the site of the injury, and making room for nutrients that are brought to the area from increased blood flow. Massaging as soon as safe after an injury minimizes the amount of scar tissue that forms, and it improves tissue structure.

Even old scars can benefit from LDM, which can help scars to become softer, smoother, and more flexible. Progress is slow, however, so it is a good idea to teach clients to self-treat daily. A combination of connective tissue massage, such as deep-tissue massage or myofascial release with LDM, produces the best results.

LOCATING INGUINAL LYMPH NODES

Lymph nodes for the abdomen and lower extremities are in the femoral triangle, bounded by the inguinal ligament and the sartorius and adductor muscles (Figure 12–1). The femoral artery is in the femoral triangle with the lymph nodes. There are two chains of lymph nodes, one near the inguinal ligament, called the horizontal or superior chain, and the other along the femoral vein, called the vertical or inferior chain. A small group of nodes, called the popliteal nodes, is near the medial knee.

These lymph nodes receive fluid from the superficial tissues of the abdomen, the lower back and gluteal regions, and the legs. Lymph from the abdominal

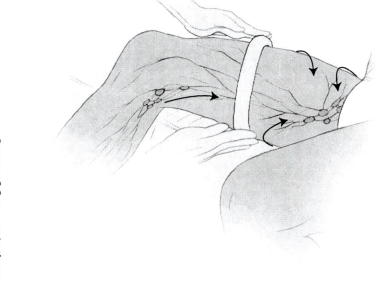

© Milady, a part of Cengage Learning.

FIGURE 12–1 Inguinal lymph nodes

region drains inferiorly, toward the inguinal nodes. Lymph from the gluteal region drains laterally around the hips to the inguinal nodes. Lymph from the lower extremities drains superiorly to the inguinal nodes. However, on the back of the thigh, lymph from the medial side drains medially, around to the front of the thigh and up to the inguinal nodes. Lymph from the lateral side of the posterior thigh drains laterally, around to the front of the thigh and up to the inguinal nodes.

From the inguinal nodes, lymph fluid drains into the iliac nodes and eventually into the lumbar trunks. The lumbar trunks also drain lymph from the pelvic organs. Other organs in the abdominal cavity have their own lymph nodes. Organ lymph nodes and the lymph nodes from the intestines eventually drain into the intestinal trunk (Table 12–1).

The lumbar trunks and the intestinal trunk join to form the **cisterna chyli**, which is the inferior end of the thoracic duct.

TABLE 12–1

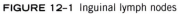

STRUCTURE	LOCATION	AFFERENTS FROM	EFFERENTS TO	REGIONS DRAINED
Cisterna chyli[1]	At the level of L1 or L2 vertebral body, between the abdominal aorta and the inferior vena cava	Intestinal trunk, right and left lumbar trunks	Thoracic duct	All of the body below the respiratory diaphragm including abdominal and pelvic organs
Intestinal trunk[2]	Left side of the abdominal aorta or between the abdominal aorta and the inferior vena cava near level of duodenum and pancreas	Union of efferent lymphatic vessels from the celiac nodes and superior mesenteric nodes	Thoracic duct via cisterna chyli or left lumbar trunk	Large and small intestines

(Continued)

STRUCTURE	LOCATION	AFFERENTS FROM	EFFERENTS TO	REGIONS DRAINED
Lumbar trunk	On the right, between the lumbar vertebrae and inferior vena cava; on the left between the lumbar vertebrae and the abdominal aorta	Lumbar chain of nodes	Thoracic duct via the cisterna chyli	Right and left halves of body below the level of the respiratory diaphragm
Lumbar nodes	Along the inferior vena cava and abdominal aorta from the aortic bifurcation to the diaphragm	Common iliac nodes; lymphatic vessels from the posterior abdominal wall and abdominal organs	Efferents form one lumbar trunk on each side	Lower limb; pelvic organs; perineum; anterior and posterior abdominal wall; kidneys; suprarenal gland; respiratory diaphragm
Common iliac nodes	Along the common iliac vessels; at the level of the body of the first sacral vertebra	External iliac nodes; internal iliac nodes	Lumbar chain of nodes	Lower limb; pelvic organs; perineum lower part of the anterior abdominal wall
External iliac nodes	Along the external iliac vessels	Superficial inguinal nodes; deep inguinal nodes; inferior epigastric nodes	Common iliac nodes	Lower limb; external genitalia; lower part of the anterior abdominal wall
Iliac nodes, internal	Along the internal iliac vessels	Lymphatic vessels from the pelvic organs	Common iliac nodes; external iliac nodes	Pelvis, perineum and gluteal region
Deep inguinal nodes	Medial side of femoral vein, inferior to the inguinal ligament	Superficial inguinal nodes; popliteal nodes	External iliac nodes	Lower limb; external genitalia; lower part of the anterior abdominal wall
Superficial inguinal nodes	Parallel and inferior to the inguinal ligament	Superficial vessels of lower limb, abdominal wall, and perineum	External iliac nodes; deep inguinal nodes	Lower abdominal wall; external genitalia; superficial parts of the lower limb
Popliteal nodes	In the popliteal fossa along the popliteal vessels	Lymph vessels that follow the anterior tibial, posterior tibial, and fibular blood vessels	Deep and superficial inguinal nodes	Leg and foot

[1]In about 25% of people the cisterna chyli is a widening at the bottom of the thoracic duct, but that doesn't exist in all individuals.

[2]Contains lymph emulsified with dietary fat.

OBSERVING AND PALPATING THE INGUINAL LYMPH NODES

Help the client lie on the table in a supine position, with the knees slightly flexed. Locate the inguinal ligament and the sartorius and rectus femoris muscles. Lymph nodes are located inferior to the inguinal ligament in the depression medial to the muscles. Rest flat fingers gently on the femoral triangle and wait a few seconds to feel the femoral pulse. Using flat fingertips, gently massage over the femoral triangle to locate the lymph nodes. Small lymph nodes that move with the skin are normal (Figure 12–2). Enlarged, tender lymph nodes indicate an infection or another disease process. Discontinue the massage and refer the client to a physician to rule out infection.

MASSAGE PROCEDURE: MASSAGING THE INGUINAL NODES, ABDOMEN AND AFFECTED LEG

Unless otherwise indicated, use stationary circles. Each circle should last 7 seconds and should be repeated for at least one minute.

Begin the massage with the client in the supine position, face up. Massage the cervical, axillary, and inguinal lymph nodes on both sides of the trunk. Massage each set of nodes for at least one minute, or until the skin and underlying tissue are softer, warmer and much more flexible.

After massaging all the lymph nodes, begin with the unaffected side of the body. Massage the vertical and horizontal chains of lymph nodes in the femoral triangle for at least a minute, until the skin and underlying tissue is softer, warmer, and able to be stretched in a larger circle. Massage the abdomen, on the unaffected side, beginning near the inguinal ligament and gradually covering the area from the inguinal ligament to the waist, from the midline to the side, as far laterally as possible without turning the client.

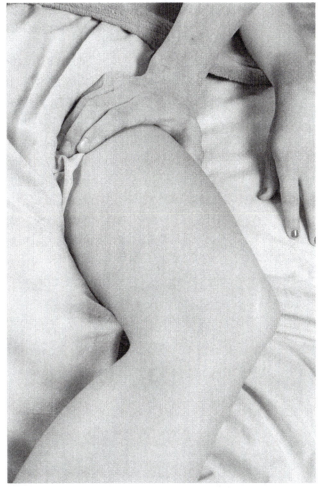

FIGURE 12-2 Locating inguinal nodes

© Milady, a part of Cengage Learning. Photography by Yanik Chauvin.

Repeat the massage of the lymph nodes and abdominal region on the affected side. Massage the lymph nodes first, and then the proximal quadrant of the trunk, from the inguinal nodes to the waist, from the midline to the side, laterally as far as possible.

Massage the leg on the affected side, beginning proximal to the nodes and working distally along the leg, covering the front, sides and back of the leg (as far as practical) down to the foot. Massage the foot and toes. Massage from the toes back up to the inguinal nodes, massaging each area for at least one minute or until the skin and underlying tissue are softer, warmer, and able to be stretched in larger circles.

Assist the client in turning over, into the prone position. Massage the gluteal region, starting proximal to the nodes and working toward the gluteal crease, the posterior midline, and the waist. Massage the back of the affected leg, beginning proximally at the gluteal crease and massaging distally, step by step, until the entire leg and foot have been massaged. Massage from the toes back to the gluteal crease again.

Finish by assisting the client to turn over to the supine position again and massage the inguinal nodes again for at least one minute.

STEP-BY-STEP

Massaging the Inguinal Nodes, Abdomen, and Affected Leg

Gather equipment and supplies. Ask the client to lie down on the massage table in the supine position, face up, and cover the client warmly. Place a small bolster under the client's knees and a small pillow under the ankle of the affected leg to be massaged.

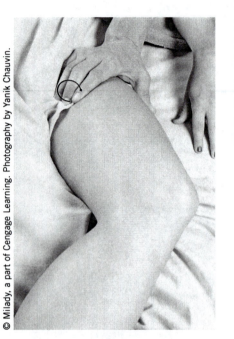

Standing at the unaffected side, locate the femoral pulse in the femoral triangle. Place fingertips on the femoral pulse, and the ulnar side of the hand and little finger along the inguinal ligament. With the hand in this position, the therapist can massage the vertical and horizontal chains of nodes at the same time. Massage the inguinal nodes for at least one minute or longer until the area is warm, soft, and the tissue stretches in larger circles.

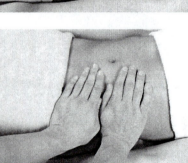

Move the hands so that the fingertips reach down the side close to the massage table, between the waist and great trochanter, with the heels of the hands near the inguinal ligament as before. Massage for one minute, moving lymph toward the inguinal nodes.

Move the hands so that the fingertips are spread along the waist, and the heels of the hands are close to the inguinal ligament. Massage as before for at least one minute, moving lymph inferiorly toward the inguinal nodes.

Place the hands over the abdomen between the inguinal ligament and navel, with the fingertips along the body's midline and the heels of the hands near the inguinal ligament. Using both hands, move the skin of the abdomen in large, slow circles, draining lymph inferiorly toward the inguinal nodes.

Massaging the Affected Lower Limb

Remember the basic elements of lymph drainage massage. Move the skin in circles, and work slowly, repeating circles six to ten times a minute. Use light pressure, from one half ounce to eight ounces of pressure per square inch. Lymph on the lower limbs drains toward the inguinal nodes.

Massage along the "side seam" of the thigh. Place the hands over the upper third of the iliotibial band, near the hip joint, and massage for about one minute.

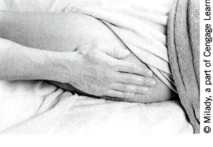
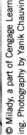

Place the hands over the middle third of the iliotibial band, and massage for one minute.

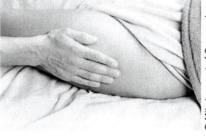
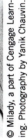

Place the hands over the lower third of the iliotibial band, near the knee, and massage for one minute.

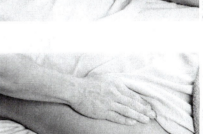

Massage along the front of the thigh from the inguinal crease to the knee. Place the hands over the upper third of the anterior thigh, inferior to the inguinal crease, covering the upper rectus femoris muscle, and massage for at least one minute, moving lymph superiorly toward the inguinal nodes.

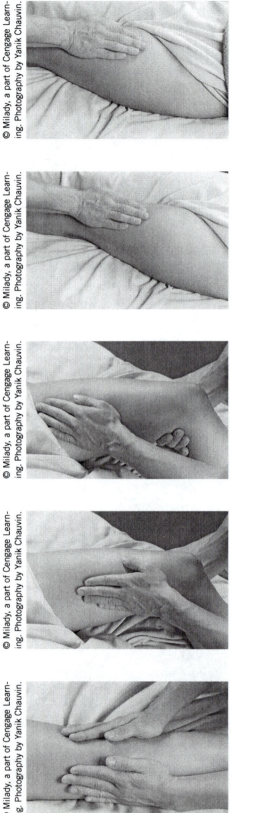

Place the hands at about the midpoint of the anterior thigh, and repeat circles for at least one minute.

Place the hands superior to the knee, at the lower third of the anterior thigh, and repeat circles for at least one minute.

Roll the knee out slightly, away from the midline, to make access to the inner thigh easier. Place the hands over the upper half of the medial thigh, and massage for at least one minute, moving fluid toward the lymph nodes.

Place hands on the medial side of the upper leg, heels of the hands near the knee crease and fingers pointing toward the inguinal nodes, over the adductor muscles. Massage for at least a minute, moving lymph fluid toward the lymph nodes.

Place the hands around the knee and use a scooping motion to move fluid toward the inguinal nodes. A "scoop" is a semicircle. Each scoop should take seven seconds, and should be repeated seven times. To do this, place one hand on each side of the knee, compress slightly, and stretch the skin in a semicircle toward the lymph nodes. Then, release the pressure and return to the point of origin.

Working from the knee to the ankle, use a scooping motion with one or both hands to move fluid toward the nodes. It will take three or four steps, repeating the movements seven times at each step, or about four minutes total for the lower leg.

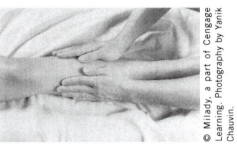

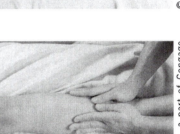

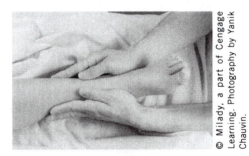

Using flat fingers, perform stationary circles around the bony protuberances of the ankles.

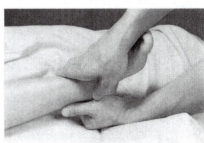

Complete stationary circles on the dorsum (top) of the foot.

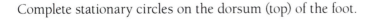

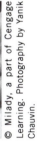

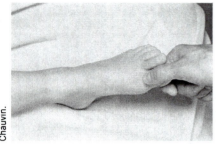

© Milady, a part of Cengage Learning. Photography by Yanik Chauvin.

Using a very slow, scooping motion with the thumb and forefinger, massage each toe seven times for about one minute per toe.

Reverse the preceding steps to work back up the leg to the inguinal nodes. Continue using slow, stationary circles or scooping movements.

Massage over the inguinal nodes using stationary circles twenty times, for about three minutes.

Help the client turn over to a prone position, and drape warmly. If the client desires, place a small pillow or rolled towel under the ankle joints.

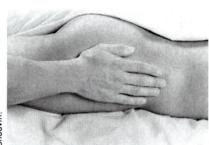

© Milady, a part of Cengage Learning. Photography by Yanik Chauvin.

Place the hands so that the heels of the hands are close to the great trochanter with the fingers pointing toward the waist, parallel to the massage table. Massage for one minute.

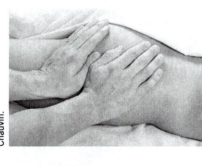

© Milady, a part of Cengage Learning. Photography by Yanik Chauvin.

Place the hands so that the heels of the hands are close to the great trochanter with the fingers pointing toward the sacrum, and massage for one minute.

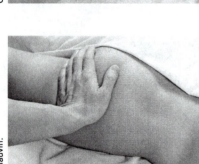

© Milady, a part of Cengage Learning. Photography by Yanik Chauvin.

Using flat hands, massage the gluteal region in a fan-shaped pattern. Place the hands so that the heels of the hands are close to the great trochanter with the fingers parallel to the gluteal crease. Massage for one minute.

Massage the lumbar region.

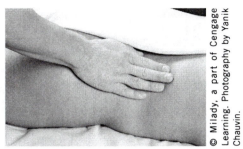

© Milady, a part of Cengage Learning. Photography by Yanik Chauvin.

Massage over the sacrum.

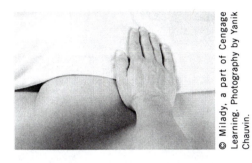

© Milady, a part of Cengage Learning. Photography by Yanik Chauvin.

Complete stationary circles over the back of the knee to open the popliteal nodes.

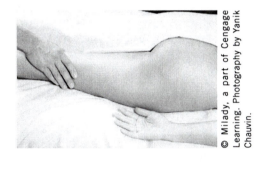

© Milady, a part of Cengage Learning. Photography by Yanik Chauvin.

Place flat hands on the upper thigh, just below the gluteal crease. Massage for one minute.

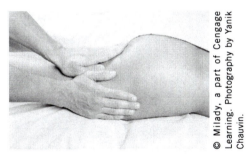

© Milady, a part of Cengage Learning. Photography by Yanik Chauvin.

Place flat hands mid-thigh, with the fingers of each hand reaching down to the massage table on each side. Massage for one minute, moving the skin in a semicircle up toward the inguinal crease and out to the sides of the thigh.

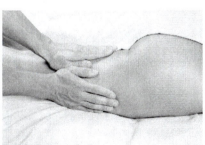

© Milady, a part of Cengage Learning. Photography by Yanik Chauvin.

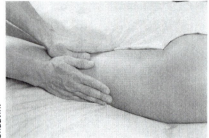

Place flat hands just above the knee on the lower thigh, with fingers reaching to the massage table on each side. Move the skin in a semicircle up toward the inguinal crease and out to the sides of the thigh.

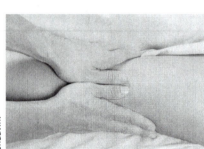

Massage the back of the knee, using stationary circles, for one minute.

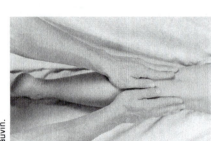

Place flat hands just below the knee on the upper calf, with fingers reaching to the massage table on each side. Move the skin in a semicircle up toward the knee and out to the sides of the calf.

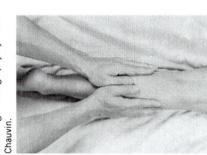

Repeat at the midpoint of the calf.

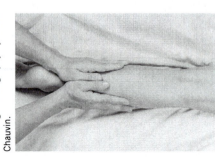

Repeat at the bottom of the calf seven times.

Using flat fingers, perform stationary circles around the bony protuberances of the ankle for one minute.

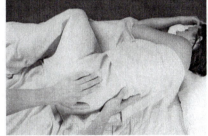

Repeat on the sole of the foot.

Reverse the preceding directions and work back up the leg to the gluteal crease.

Help the client turn over into a supine position. Drape warmly. Finish the lower quadrant by massaging over the inguinal nodes again in 20 circles.

Help the client into the fetal position to stretch the lower back.

Then, help the client sit. Use percussion or neck and shoulder massage to invigorate the client. Stand next to client as the client climbs off the massage table to prevent falling. If the client is very groggy, walk with the client, offer water, turn on the lights, open windows, and so on, to help the client become fully alert. Do not allow a client to leave until the client is fully awake and able to drive safely.

13

Abdominal Massage: Stimulating the Deep Circulation of Lymph

Themotility of abdominopelvic organs and improve breathing, which are two forces that stimulate the deep circulation of lymph.

The purpose of abdominal massage is to enhance the motility of abdominopelvic organs and improve breathing, which are two forces that stimulate the deep circulation of lymph.

Even at rest, the body is constantly moving. The heart continually beats, creating a rhythmic movement of blood throughout the entire body. Breathing goes on 24 hours a day. Abdominal peristalsis is a wave-like rhythmical contraction of the intestines that continues throughout the day. In addition, there are other continuous movements such as the cranial motion, secretion of hormones, the lymphatic pump, which is the wave-like contraction of lymph vessels, and small movements such as blinking of the eyes. On a microscopic level, there is the movement of fluid across membranes including blood vessels, lymph vessels and cell membranes, and the migration of microscopic cells such as white blood cells in blood, lymph and tissue fluid.

Inhibition of these natural movements negatively affects the deep circulation of lymph. For instance, breathing has a significant effect on the lymph propulsion. The thoracic duct is squeezed on inhalation, which forces lymph fluid out of the thoracic duct into the jugular and subclavian veins. The deeper the breath and the more the lungs fill, the more fluid is forced into the jugular and subclavian veins from the thoracic duct. This creates a partial vacuum in the thoracic duct, so that, upon exhalation, more fluid is pulled from abdominal lymph trunks into the thoracic duct.

Upon inhalation, the diaphragm moves inferiorly, displacing abdominal organs and increasing pressure in the abdomen. In response to the contraction of the diaphragm, abdominal organs move inferiorly and anteriorly, and then back up into resting position upon exhalation. As the diaphragm contracts, it pulls on lung connective tissue, creating more volume for air. As the diaphragm relaxes, it compresses the lungs and relaxes pressure on the abdominal organs.

The organs in the abdomen, although moveable, are held in place by a variety of structures. Tendons connect organs to each other and to the back wall of the abdomen. The folds of the peritoneum keep the organs in place relative to each other and relative to the abdominal wall. The mesentery is an extension of the peritoneum which loosely connects the intestines to the back wall of the abdomen. Organs and connective tissue are lubricated by tissue fluid. The organs and folds of the mesentery should move freely in response to the rhythm of diaphragmatic movement and abdominal peristalsis. Each organ has its own lymph nodes and lymph vessels which are massaged by the continuous movement of the diaphragm and abdominopelvic organs.

Movement of abdominal organs can be inhibited due to scar tissue because of injury, accident, surgery, inactivity, infections, or overweight, all of which cause inflammation. In the inflammatory process, fibers are laid down in the inflamed area to wall off infectious organisms and to rebuild damaged tissue. As a result, the tissue changes in texture, becoming coarser and less flexible. Layers of tissue that should slide over each other in response to abdominal rhythms instead become glued together, further limiting movement. This fascial binding, called an adhesion, causes connective tissue to harden like an inflexible girdle. This inhibits the movement of abdominal organs and the circulation of lymph.

Therefore, the purpose of abdominal massage is to remove or reduce fascial binding, which will enhance the motility of abdominopelvic organs and improve breathing. This is done by carefully massaging the abdomen, layer by tissue layer,

Purpose of Abdominal Massage

- Stimulate deep lymph circulation
- Release abdominal adhesions
- Promote motility of abdominopelvic organs
- Relax breathing muscles
- Stimulate abdominal peristalsis
- Increase lymph flow from the abdomen into the cisterna chyli and thoracic duct

stretching any adhesions that are found. It requires knowledge of abdominopelvic anatomy and experience with connective tissue massage. The therapist will end the massage with wave-like compressions that have been shown to increase lymph flow through the thoracic duct into the central veins, and to increase the number of leukocytes flowing through the duct.

In order to avoid harming any client, the therapist must patiently and slowly work through each connective tissue layer using touch that is within the client's comfort range. Clients must participate in their therapy, providing feedback for the therapist during the massage. The therapist should communicate clearly what will happen during the massage, and what is expected from the client. The therapist should also be willing to listen to the client's feedback, and change massage techniques or halt the massage if necessary.

The massage should never be painful; if the client reports experiencing pain, the therapist should stop working and try to assess the reason for the pain. If it isn't due to excessive pressure by the massage therapist, is the pain in a muscle that can be identified? Does the pain improve with gentle massage? If the therapist can't identify the reason for the pain, and it doesn't improve with gentle massage, the massage should be terminated and the client referred to his/her physician.

Contraindications

The same contraindications that apply to lymphatic drainage massage also apply to abdominal massage. There are additional contraindications for this area of the body. Abdominal massage should not be given to a pregnant woman, or to anyone who has had a recent injury to the abdomen or pelvis, recent abdominal or pelvic surgery or infection, or chronic or severe pain that has not been examined by a physician. Do not give abdominal massage to anyone with a history of abdominal hernia unless the client's physician has approved the massage.

STRUCTURE

The abdominopelvic cavity is a hollow area formed by the ribs, lumbar spine and the pelvis. Outside the skeletal structure of the abdominopelvic cavity are skin, muscles, connective tissue and membranes that wrap around the abdominal contents like layers of fabric wrapped around a balloon, surrounding the cavity which contains the abdominal and pelvic organs.

Contraindications to Abdominal Lymphatic Drainage Massage

- Pregnancy
- Undiagnosed chronic and/or severe abdominal pain
- Infection, illness
- Severe or chronic low back pain that is undiagnosed
- Ruptured vertebral disk
- Recent injury or surgery
- Heart disease, kidney disease, liver disease, heart attack or heart surgery in the last year
- Skin disease (contagious disease or one that might be irritated by massage)
- Blood-thinning medications such as coumadin, or a blood disease such as hemophilia
- Medical implants such as a stent
- Difficulty communicating clearly, for instance a young child, a deaf person, someone who speaks a different language or anyone who has difficulty speaking, for instance, after a stroke

Under the skin is a layer of fascia containing lymph vessels and fat cells. Beneath this superficial fascia is a layer of connective tissue which contains the muscles that form the walls of the abdomen. Contained inside the wrapping of muscles, connective tissue and the skeleton are the abdominopelvic organs. Although they are closely packed, they are lubricated by the fluid in the abdomen, which enables them to move as the diaphragm contracts and presses down on them. The deep muscles of the abdominopelvic cavity include the psoas major and minor, iliacus, and the levator ani. The levator ani muscles are called the diaphragm of the pelvis; they form the floor of the pelvis and support the pelvic organs.

The general procedure is to perform lymph drainage massage to the supraclavicular nodes, infraclavicular nodes, and axillary and inguinal lymph nodes. Then perform lymph drainage massage on the four quadrants of the abdomen, moving lymph toward the appropriate lymph nodes.

Next, massage the superficial fascia and the layers of connective tissue which contain the muscles that form the walls of the abdomen—the quadratus lumborum, thoracolumbar fascia, internal and external oblique muscles, transversus muscle and rectus abdominis.

The therapist will then massage the middle layers of the abdomen, stretching layers of connective tissue under the lower ribs, inside the iliac bowl, along the pubic ridge, and massaging the area of the large and small intestines, penetrating to the psoas muscles. End the massage with lymphatic compressions on the abdomen, creating a wave-like motion in the abdominal tissue.[1,2]

Skeletal Structure

The skeletal framework of the abdomen consists of the lower rib cage, the ilium, ischium, pubis and sacrum, and the lower part of the vertebral column. These bony structures do not completely surround and protect abdominopelvic contents, but they provide protection for important organs including the liver

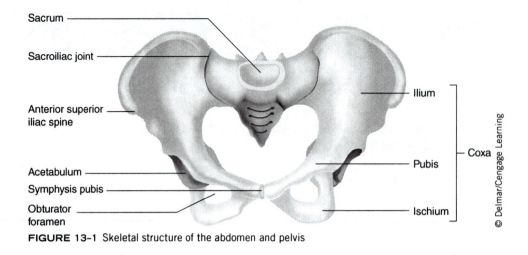

Sacrum

Sacroiliac joint

Anterior superior
iliac spine

Ilium

Coxa

Acetabulum

Pubis

Symphysis pubis

Obturator
foramen

Ischium

© Delmar/Cengage Learning

FIGURE 13-1 Skeletal structure of the abdomen and pelvis

and kidneys. These bones also provide the structure which supports the muscles, tendons, ligaments and fascia that surround, protect and connect the abdominopelvic organs.

Lower Ribs

There are 12 sets of ribs. The upper seven ribs are connected to the thoracic spine in the back, and to the sternum via costal cartilage in the front. The next three ribs on each side connect to the costal cartilage of the ribs above them, rather than connecting to the sternum. The bottom two ribs, called floating ribs, are not attached to any skeletal structure in the front of the trunk. The lower ribs, sternum and xiphoid process are the sites of the attachments of the diaphragm muscle, which forms the roof of the abdominopelvic cavity.

Lumbar Spine

The lumbar spine consists of five very large vertebrae which are the attachment sites for the psoas and quadratus lumborum muscles. The psoas can be palpated in the abdomen, as it originates on the anterior surfaces of the lumbar vertebrae and transverse processes. The psoas descends through the abdomen and connects to the lesser trochanter on the femur.

The quadratus lumborum muscles connect to the posterior surfaces of the transverse processes of the lumbar spine, as well as the lower ribs and the iliac crest. The quadratus lumborum, psoas major, erector spinae and thoracolumbar fascia form the back wall of the abdomen.

Ilium

The ilium is the wide wing-shaped part of the hip bone. It is easily palpated. The iliac crest is the high point of the ilium, the part of the hip that forms the waist. It runs from the anterior superior iliac spine in the front (the most anterior part of the ilium) to the posterior superior iliac spine in the back (the most posterior part of the ilium), near the sacrum. The iliac tubercle is the widest point of the ilium, and is located posterior to the anterior iliac spine.

MUSCLES OF THE ABDOMINAL WALL AND RESPIRATION

Muscles of the Abdominal Wall

Muscle	Origin	Insertion	Function
External oblique	Lower eight ribs	Iliac crest, Anterior rectus sheath	Compresses abdominal contents
Internal oblique	Iliac crest	Costal cartilage, lower three or four ribs	Compresses abdominal contents
Transversus abdominis	Iliac crest, cartilage of lower six ribs	Xiphoid cartilage, linea alba	Compresses abdominal contents
Rectus abdominis	Crest of pubis, pubic symphysis	Cartilage of 5th, 6th, 7th rib	Flexes vertebral column, assists in compressing abdominal wall

Muscles of Respiration

Muscle	Origin	Insertion	Function
Diaphragm	Xiphoid process, costal cartilages, lumbar vertebrae	Central tendon	Increases vertical diameter of thorax
External intercostals	Lower border of rib	Upper border of rib below	Draws adjacent ribs together
Internal intercostals	Ridge on inner surface of rib	Upper border of rib below	Draws adjacent ribs together
Quadratus lumborum	Iliac crest	Last rib and upper four lumbar vertebrae	Flexes trunk laterally

FIGURE 13–2 Muscles of the abdominal wall and respiration

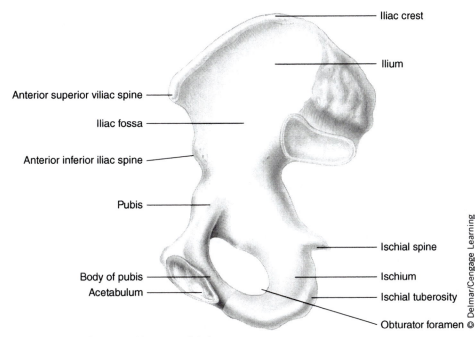

FIGURE 13–3 Right coxal bone, medial view

Pubis Symphysis and Pubic Ridge

The pubic ridge can be found by palpating inferiorly from the navel until the ridge can be felt. The pubic crest consists of the pubic bones connected by the cartilaginous pubis symphysis, which forms a rigid joint between the pubic bones.

Inguinal Ligament

The inguinal ligament is an extension of the aponeurosis of the external oblique muscle. It extends from the anterior superior iliac spine to the pubic bone. The connective tissue of the external oblique muscle is continuous with the connective tissue of the serratus anterior muscle and the rhomboid muscles. This forms a continuous band of connective tissue from the upper thoracic spine, wrapping around the rib cage, to the ilium and thence to the pubic bones via the inguinal ligament.

ORGANS

Except for the large intestine and sometimes the bladder or uterus, the internal organs are not easy to palpate unless pathology is present. If the liver or stomach is easily palpable, for instance, the client may have a serious disorder and should be examined by a physician. The uterus is easily palpable during pregnancy, but this is a contraindication for deep abdominal massage. If the uterus can be felt and the client is not pregnant, end the massage and refer the client for examination. Any masses in the abdomen which can be palpated and which are obviously not muscle or fascia should be noted, and the client referred to a physician for diagnosis.

Abdominal Aorta

To find the abdominal aorta, place fingertips on the midline of the trunk, above the navel. If the pulse can't be felt above the navel, try to find it on the left side of the navel or slightly below and left (the client's left).

Stomach

The stomach is located on the client's left side, protected by the rib cage. During inhalation, the stomach moves downward in the abdomen and can sometimes be felt along the margin of the ribs. If the stomach feels hard or enlarged, the client should be referred to his or her physician.

Spleen

The spleen is behind the stomach, protected by the rib cage and not palpable by the massage therapist.

Liver and Gallbladder

The liver and gallbladder are located on the client's right side, protected by the ribs, although the lower margin of the liver may be palpated when it moves

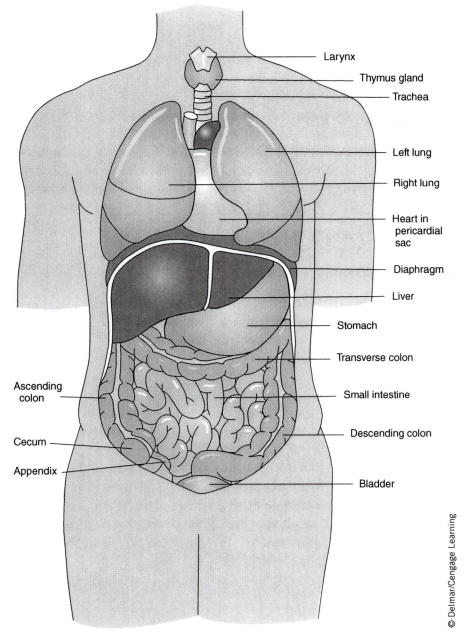

Larynx

Thymus gland

Trachea

Left lung

Right lung

Heart in pericardial sac

Diaphragm

Liver

Stomach

Transverse colon

Ascending colon

Small intestine

Descending colon

Cecum

Appendix

Bladder

© Delmar/Cengage Learning

FIGURE 13-4 Thoracic and abdominopelvic cavities

downward into the abdominal cavity on inspiration. On exhalation of the breath, the liver moves upward under the ribs. If the liver is easily palpable and hard or enlarged, the client should be referred to his/her physician for examination.

Small Intestine

If the therapist is working slowly and carefully, the small intestines slide out of the way and are not usually palpable unless full or very active. The therapist may be able to feel movement in the small intestines if they are full of liquid or gas. The ascending and transverse colon are not usually palpable. However, the descending colon can often be felt if it is full. If the therapist is working quickly with heavy pressure, the intestines can be pinched between the therapist's fingers and bone, causing a bruise or other damage.

Bladder

The bladder is posterior to and partly covered by the pubic ridge. It isn't easy to palpate unless it is very full or scarred, and pressure on a full bladder is uncomfortable for the client.

Reproductive Organs

The uterus is not usually palpable unless it is scarred, has palpable cysts, or the client is pregnant. It is located posterior to the urinary bladder and is larger than the urinary bladder. Pregnancy is a contraindication for abdominal massage.

MUSCLES AND FASCIA

Rectus Abdominis

To locate the rectus abdominis muscle, place fingers on either side of the xiphoid process, below the margin of the ribs. As your client performs slight crunches, palpate the body of the muscle down to the pubic ridge.

External Oblique

Place your hands across the trunk on the (client's) right side of the abdomen, between the lateral ribs and the iliac crest. Ask your client to move the right shoulder toward the left hip. You should be able to feel the external oblique muscle contract. Repeat on the opposite side. The origin is on the lower eight ribs, interwoven with the serratus anterior muscle. The fibers of the muscle run inferiorly toward the insertion on the anterior iliac crest and the abdominal aponeurosis. The external oblique muscle flexes the trunk when both sides contract. If only one side is contracted, the muscle laterally flexes the trunk and rotates the spine toward the opposite side.

Internal Oblique

The origin of the internal oblique muscle is on the lateral inguinal ligament, the crest of the ilium, and the thoracolumbar fascia. The fibers of the internal oblique muscle run obliquely to the external oblique muscle fibers, toward the insertion on the lower three ribs and the abdominal aponeurosis. The action of the internal oblique muscle is to flex the trunk (both sides contracted) and if only one side is contracted, laterally flex the trunk and rotate the spine to the same side.

Transversus Abdominis

The origin of this muscle is on the cartilage of the seventh through twelfth ribs, lumbar fascia, and the iliac crest and inguinal ligament. The insertion is on the linea alba and the xiphoid cartilage. The transversus abdominis muscle compresses the abdominal contents, contributing to the shape of the body.

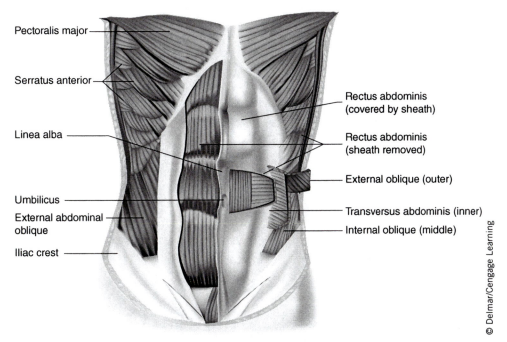

Pectoralis major

Serratus anterior

Linea alba

Umbilicus

External abdominal oblique

Iliac crest

Rectus abdominis (covered by sheath)

Rectus abdominis (sheath removed)

External oblique (outer)

Transversus abdominis (inner)

Internal oblique (middle)

© Delmar/Cengage Learning

FIGURE 13–5 External and internal oblique muscles

Diaphragm

The diaphragm originates on the first, second and third lumbar vertebrae, the lower six costal cartilages, the inner surface of the lower six ribs, and the inner surface of the xiphoid process of the sternum. The insertion of this muscular membranous partition is on the central tendon, which connects to the fascia of the lungs. When the diaphragm contracts, it flattens, pulling down on the fascia of the lungs, which increases the volume of lungs and draws air in through the respiratory tract.

Psoas Major

The origin is on the anterior aspect of the transverse processes of the lumbar vertebrae, the anterior aspect of the bodies of the T12-L5 vertebrae, and the disks of each lumbar vertebra. The insertion is on the lesser trochanter of the femur. The psoas muscle is a hip flexor, but also helps to create the curve of the lumbar spine. When the legs are fixed, tightening the psoas muscle pulls the spine toward the legs, as in a sit-up exercise.

Iliacus

The origin is along the upper two thirds of the iliac fossa, and the insertion is into the lesser trochanter of the femur. The iliacus muscle is also a hip flexor, and tilts the iliac crest forward and down.

Quadratus Lumborum

The origin is on the iliac crest, and the insertion is into the border of the last rib (T12) and the transverse processes of the L1-L4 vertebrae. The quadratus lumborum muscle flexes the lower back laterally when one side is tightened, and extends the lower back when both sides are tightened. The quadratus lumborum helps to stabilize the lower back, opposes the psoas and iliacus, hikes the ilium and flattens the low back. It is smaller than the psoas and more likely to hurt if the psoas is overly contracted.

Piriformis

The origin is on the anterior (pelvic) surface of the sacrum and the insertion is on the superior border of the great trochanter. The piriformis muscle laterally rotates the femur.

Levator Ani

This muscle forms the floor of the pelvis, originating on the pubis and ischium, and inserting on the anterior surface of the coccyx, the levator ani of the opposite side, and the sides of the rectum. It supports and slightly raises the pelvic floor and constricts the lower end of the rectum and vagina.

FASCIA

The fascia of the abdominal muscles is a sheet of fibrous tissue that unites the muscles to form a sphere that contains the abdominal contents and affects posture,

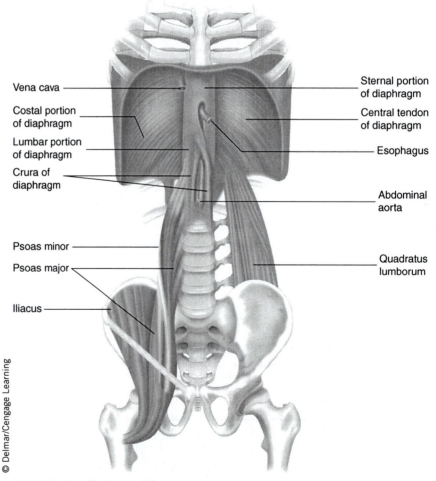

© Delmar/Cengage Learning

FIGURE 13–6 Diaphragm, illiopsoas and quadratus lumborum

movement, and breathing. The central tendon of the diaphragm connects to the fascia of the lungs so that when the diaphragm contracts, the lungs are pulled downwards, pulling air into the lungs. The right and left crus of the diaphragm connect with the fascia of the psoas, which bridges the lower back and the lower limbs. The fascia of the psoas muscle connects with the fascia of the quadratus lumborum, which also connects the lower ribs with the ilium.

The girdle muscles, external oblique, internal oblique, and transversus abdominis muscles form three layers of muscles that connect in the back to the thoracolumbar fascia, and in the front to the abdominal aponeurosis and linea alba. These muscles also connect the lower ribs with the ilium.

Because all of these muscles are connected to each other by means of fascia, contracture in one or a few of these muscles affects all of them, and affects posture, movement, and breathing, as well as causing symptoms in the organs contained within the muscular sphere.

NODES AND VESSELS

All the lymph from the superficial and deep circulation in the lower extremities and lymph from the pelvic organs drains to the inguinal nodes, and then travels through the iliac nodes to the lumbar trunks. Lymph from the abdomen and abdominal organs drains to local lymph nodes, named for their locations or for the organs that they drain, and then to the intestinal trunk or directly to the thoracic duct. Lymph from the intestines and mesentery drains into the intestinal trunk. The intestinal and lumbar trunks join to form the cisterna chyli, the lower end of the thoracic duct.

Some organs drain in several directions. The upper stomach, for instance, drains in a different direction than the lower stomach, but all the gastric lymph fluid eventually winds up in the thoracic duct. From the thoracic duct, lymph is drained into the subclavian vein or internal jugular vein.

STRUCTURE	LOCATION	AFFERENTS FROM	EFFERENTS TO	REGIONS DRAINED
Thoracic duct	Between the esophagus and the thoracic vertebrae	Lumbar and intestinal trunks	Left subclavian or left internal jugular vein	All lymphatics below the diaphragm, left side of the trunk above the diaphragm, left arm, left side of the head and neck
Cisterna chyli1 (junction of lumbar trunks and intestinal trunk)	Level with L1 or L2 vertebra between the abdominal aorta and the inferior vena cava	Intestinal trunk, right and left lumbar trunks	Thoracic duct	All of the body below the respiratory diaphragm including abdominal and pelvic organs
Intestinal trunk2	On the left of the abdominal aorta near level of pancreas	Union of efferent lymphatic vessels from the celiac nodes and superior mesenteric nodes	Thoracic duct	Large and small intestines

(Continued)

STRUCTURE	LOCATION	AFFERENTS FROM	EFFERENTS TO	REGIONS DRAINED
Lumbar trunk	On the right, between the lumbar vertebrae and inferior vena cava, on the left between the lumbar vertebrae and the abdominal aorta	Lumbar chain of nodes	Thoracic duct via the cisterna chyli	Right and left halves of body below the level of the respiratory diaphragm
Lumbar nodes	Along the inferior vena cava and abdominal aorta from the aortic bifurcation to the diaphragm	Common iliac nodes; lymphatic vessels from the posterior abdominal wall and abdominal organs	Efferents form one lumbar trunk on each side	Lower limb; pelvic organs; perineum; anterior and posterior abdominal wall; kidneys; suprarenal gland; respiratory diaphragm
Common iliac nodes	Along the common iliac vessels; at the level of the body of the first sacral vertebra	External iliac nodes, internal iliac nodes	Lumbar chain of nodes	Lower limb; pelvic organs, perineum, lower part of the anterior abdominal wall
External iliac nodes	Along the external iliac vessels	Superficial inguinal nodes; deep inguinal nodes; inferior epigastric nodes	Common iliac nodes	Lower limb; external genitalia; lower part of the anterior abdominal wall
Iliac nodes, internal	Along the internal iliac vessels	Lymphatic vessels from the pelvic organs	Common iliac nodes, external iliac nodes	Pelvis, perineum and gluteal region
colic nodes, middle	along the course of the middle colic vessels	peripheral nodes located along the attachment of the mesentery	superior mesenteric nodes	transverse colon
colic nodes, right	along the course of the right colic vessels	peripheral nodes located along the marginal a.	superior mesenteric nodes	ascending colon, cecum
cystic node	near the neck of the gall bladder	lymphatic vessels of the gall bladder	hepatic nodes	gall bladder
gastric nodes, left	on the lesser curvature of the stomach, along the course of the left gastric vessels	lymphatic vessels from the lesser curvature of the stomach	celiac nodes	lesser curvature of the stomach
gastric nodes, right	on the lesser curvature of the stomach, along the course of the right gastric vessels	lymphatic vessels from the lesser curvature of the stomach	celiac nodes	lesser curvature of the stomach
gastro-omental nodes, left	on the greater curvature of the stomach, along the left gastro-omental vessels	lymphatic vessels from the greater curvature of the stomach	splenic nodes	left half of the greater curvature of the stomach

(Continued)

STRUCTURE	LOCATION	AFFERENTS FROM	EFFERENTS TO	REGIONS DRAINED
gastro-omental nodes, right	on the greater curvature of the stomach, along the right gastro-omental vessels	lymphatic vessels from the greater curvature of the stomach	pyloric nodes	greater curvature of the stomach
hepatic nodes	along the course of the common hepatic a.	right gastric nodes, pyloric nodes	celiac nodes	liver and gall bladder; extrahepatic biliary apparatus; respiratory diaphragm; head of pancreas and duodenum
ileocolic nodes	along the origin and terminal end of the ileocolic vessels	peripheral nodes located along the attachment of the mesentery	superior mesenteric nodes	ileum, cecum, appendix
inferior mesenteric nodes	around the root of the inferior mesenteric a.	peripheral nodes located along the marginal a.	lumbar chain of nodes, superior mesenteric nodes	distal 1/3 of the transverse colon, descending colon, sigmoid colon, rectum
intercostal nodes	near the heads of the ribs	lymphatic vessels from the intercostal space	cisterna chyli/thoracic duct, jugulosubclavian duct	intercostal space and posterolateral thoracic wall
lateral aortic nodes (lumbar nodes)	along the inferior vena cava and abdominal aorta from the aortic bifurcation to the aortic hiatus of the diaphragm	common iliac nodes; lymphatic vessels from the posterior abdominal wall and viscera	efferents form one lumbar trunk on each side	lower limb; pelvic organs; perineum; anterior and posterior abdominal wall; kidney; suprarenal gland; respiratory diaphragm
left gastric nodes	on the lesser curvature of the stomach, along the course of the left gastric vessels	lymphatic vessels from the lesser curvature of the stomach	celiac nodes	lesser curvature of the stomach
left gastro-omental nodes	on the greater curvature of the stomach, along the left gastro-omental vessels	lymphatic vessels from the greater curvature of the stomach	splenic nodes	left half of the greater curvature of the stomach
mesenteric nodes	along the vasa recta and branches of the superior mesenteric a. between the leaves of peritoneum forming the mesentery	peripheral nodes located along the attachment of the mesentery	superior mesenteric nodes	small intestine
mesenteric nodes, inferior	around the root of the inferior mesenteric a.	peripheral nodes located along the marginal a.	lumbar chain of nodes, superior mesenteric nodes	distal 1/3 of the transverse colon, descending colon, sigmoid colon, rectum
mesenteric nodes, superior	along the course of the superior mesenteric a.	mesenteric nodes, ileocolic nodes, right colic nodes, middle colic nodes	celiac nodes, intestinal lymph trunk	gut and viscera supplied by the superior mesenteric a.

(Continued)

STRUCTURE	LOCATION	AFFERENTS FROM	EFFERENTS TO	REGIONS DRAINED
middle colic nodes	along the course of the middle colic vessels	peripheral nodes located along the attachment of the mesentery	superior mesenteric nodes	transverse colon
pancreaticoduodenal nodes	along the pancreaticoduodenal arcade of vessels	lymphatic vessels from the duodenum and pancreas	pyloric nodes	duodenum and head of the pancreas
pancreaticosplenic nodes	along the splenic vessels	lymphatic vessels from the pancreas and greater curvature of the stomach	celiac nodes	neck, body and tail of the pancreas; left half of the greater curvature of the stomach
paracardial nodes	around the esophagogastric junction	lymphatic vessels of the fundus and cardia of the stomach	left gastric nodes	fundus and cardia of the stomach
phrenic nodes	on the thoracic surface of the respiratory diaphragm	lymphatic vessels from the diaphragm, liver and thoracic wall	lumbar nodes, posterior mediastinal nodes	superior surface of the liver, respiratory diaphragm
pyloric nodes	near the termination of the gastroduodenal a.	pancreaticoduodenal nodes	hepatic nodes	head of pancreas and duodenum; right half of greater curvature of stomach
right colic nodes	along the course of the right colic vessels	peripheral nodes located along the marginal a.	superior mesenteric nodes	ascending colon, cecum
right gastric nodes	on the lesser curvature of the stomach, along the course of the right gastric vessels	lymphatic vessels from the lesser curvature of the stomach	celiac nodes	lesser curvature of the stomach
right gastro-omental nodes	on the greater curvature of the stomach, along the right gastro-omental vessels	lymphatic vessels from the greater curvature of the stomach	pyloric nodes	greater curvature of the stomach
sacral nodes	along the course of the lateral sacral aa.	lymphatic vessels from the pelvic viscera	common iliac nodes	prostate gland, uterus, vagina, rectum, posterior pelvic wall
spleen	in the abdominal cavity below the left dome of the diaphragm, anterior to the left kidney	splenic brs. of the splenic a.	splenic v.	filters blood by phagocytosis; produces T & B-lymphocytes
superior mesenteric nodes	along the course of the superior mesenteric a.	mesenteric nodes, ileocolic nodes, right colic nodes, middle colic nodes	celiac nodes, intestinal lymph trunk	gut and viscera supplied by the superior mesenteric a.

[1]In about 25% of people the cisterna chyli is a widening at the bottom of the thoracic duct, but that doesn't exist in all individuals.

[2]Contains lymph emulsified with dietary fat

MedCharts Anatomy by Thomas R. Gest and Jaye Schlesinger Published by ILOC, Inc., New York. Copyright © 1995. Lymph flow of the digestive tract Rehabilitation Oncology, 2002 by Feltman, Barbara, Petterborg, Larry http://anatomy.uams.edu/anatomyhtml/lymph_abdomen.html, accessed February, 2010

FIGURE 13-7 Lymph node chart

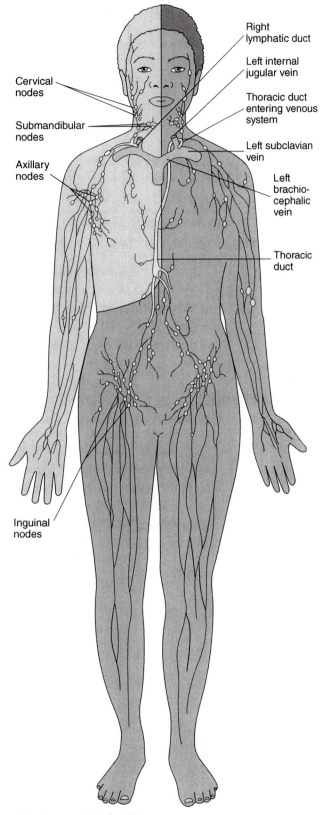

FIGURE 13–8 Lymph nodes

Outline of Abdominal Massage

With the client lying supine on the massage table, begin by rocking the abdomen gently until the client relaxes and the entire body rocks freely.

Massage the lymph nodes. Massage each set of nodes for at least a minute, until the tissue changes and becomes softer, warmer and stretches in a larger circle.

1. Supraclavicular nodes
2. Infraclavicular nodes
3. Axillary nodes
4. Inguinal nodes

Perform lymph drainage massage on the four quadrants of the abdomen, moving lymph toward the appropriate nodes.

1. Upper right quadrant, moving lymph toward the right axilla
2. Upper left quadrant, moving lymph toward the left axilla
3. Lower right quadrant, moving lymph toward the right inguinal nodes
4. Lower left quadrant, moving lymph toward the left inguinal nodes

Massage the Superficial Muscles and Connective Tissue

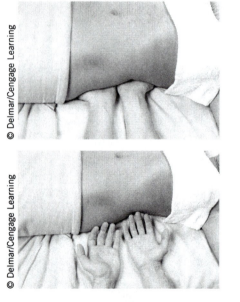

© Delmar/Cengage Learning

Slide your hands under the client's lower back, put your fingers into the proximal lamina groove (a depression along the spine), hook them into the thoracolumbar fascia and erector spinae muscle, and apply gentle traction. Hold the stretch until you feel a release. Work up and down the lumbar fascia tissue from sacrum to T10 vertebra.

Slide your hands under the client until the sacroiliac joint canbe felt. Hook your fingers into the medial side of the joint and apply gentle traction. Hold for a few seconds.

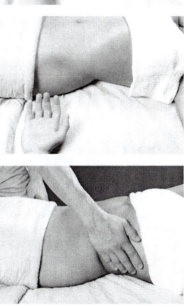

Stretch the serratus anterior and external oblique muscles. Reach across the client's trunk, and place your fingertips between the scapula and ribs. Pull the skin to the limit of the stretch, and hold until the tissue stretches further. Work along the fibers of the serratus anterior and external oblique muscles, following the band of fascia to the margin of the abdominal aponeurosis tendon.

Stretch the internal oblique muscle from its origin on the thoracolumbar fascia and iliac crest to the abdominalaponeurosis tendon and the lower ribs.

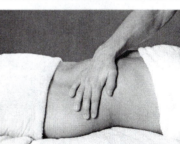

Start at the lumbar fascia tissue, and stretch the transversusmuscle around the waist to the abdominal aponeurosis tendon.

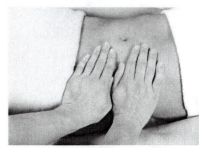

Stretch the edges of the rectus abdominis muscle, and work from center up to the sternum, and then down to the pubisbone on each edge of the muscle.

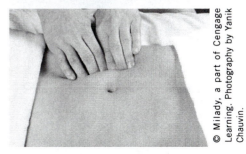

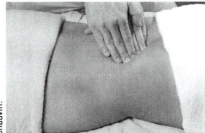

© Milady, a part of Cengage Learning. Photography by Yanik Chauvin.

Stretch the tissue under the ribs, using a fan shaped movement, working along costal margin. Turn hands palms up and stretch tissue along the interior surface of the lower ribs.

Stretch the Deeper Connective Tissue

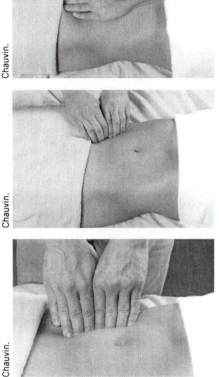

© Milady, a part of Cengage Learning. Photography by Yanik Chauvin.

Starting at the navel, palpate inferiorly until the pubic ridgecan be felt. Use stiff fingers to stretch the tissue along the pubicridge.

© Milady, a part of Cengage Learning. Photography by Yanik Chauvin.

Slide fingertips from anterior iliac spine into the bowl of the hipalong the fibers of the iliacus in the direction of the sacrum.

© Milady, a part of Cengage Learning. Photography by Yanik Chauvin.

Using paired hands, spiral gently into abdominal tissue until anobstruction is met. Rock gently in and out of the obstruction, stretching the tissue until the obstruction "disappears." Stopinstantly if any area is painful. Work very slowly, clockwise around the abdomen, covering all the tissue from the ribs inferiorly to the inguinal ligament and pubic ridge.

Locate Deeper Muscles

When abdomen is completely relaxed and soft, and client reports there is no tenderness or pain, it is time to work more deeply in the abdomen, very carefully and slowly.

Locate the psoas muscle by palpating beneath the edge of the rectus abdominis muscle about the level of the navel. Gently rock the tips of your fingers, as if you are moving the intestines aside as you move more deeply into the abdomen. Search for a strap of muscle parallel to the lumbar spine. To confirm that it is the correct muscle, keep your fingers on the strap of muscle and ask the client to flex his or her hip by drawing the heel closer to the buttocks. The psoas muscle will contract. Apply steady but gentle pressure to the muscle and ask the client to repeat the motion of sliding the heel a few inches toward the buttocks and then extending the leg again, until the movement is smooth and easy.

Locate the sacroiliac joint by sliding along the iliacus muscle posteriorly and inferiorly toward the sacrum until the edge of the sacrum can be felt. Slide over the edge of the sacrum, in an angle toward the rectum, and ask your client to rotate the femur by rolling the leg laterally and back to neutral. The rotator muscles will contract.

Pumping the Cisterna Chyli

Gently rock the abdomen until the client's entire body relaxes and rocks freely. Place your hands on the abdomen between the navel and the ribs, fingers pointing toward the midline of the trunk. Sink your fingers into the abdomen gently and then scoop in and up, as if stroking upward along the spinal column. Repeat in waves for at least a minute.

Finish by sitting down, sliding one hand under the client's sacrum and holding one hand on the client's lower abdomen. Sit up straight, with both feet on the floor, and breathe slowly. Ask the client to breathe slowly and to report when he or she can feel heat connecting between the therapist's hands.

NOTES

This is an intense massage. The therapist should proceed slowly and cautiously, and it should not hurt. If there seem to be a lot of adhesions, the work may have to be done over several sessions. There is no reason to hurry this work, and in fact, the client will benefit more if the therapist is willing to work slowly over several sessions.

After this work, the client may feel a little sore the next day, as if he or she had been working out at the gym. Alternating hot and cold packs to the lower back and abdomen is recommended.

Work this intense may trigger emotional release. Let the client guide the work; if the client doesn't want to continue because it is emotionally intense, change to another form of massage for the rest of the session. When you touch an area that has been hurt by injury, surgery, infections or treatments such as radiation, the client may suddenly experience the feelings that he or she had at the time of the original problem. It can take the client by surprise, to suddenly feel that way again. Reassure the client that it happens to others also, and that the feelings will go away. It's just a memory.

Energetic and Mind-Body Effects of Lymph Drainage Massage

Lymph drainage massage has many beneficial effects beyond the physiological processes. It affects clients on many levels. The deep relaxation LDM achieves in a conducive setting can lead both client and therapist into meditative states, with all the attendant benefits of meditation. For this mind-body work, the success of the session depends on the setting, the connection between the therapist and the client, and the work performed.

ESTABLISHING THE PROPER SETTING

The setting must feel safe to both therapist and client. Privacy must be insured, and the room should be quiet, dim, and serene. Music, if used, should be unobtrusive. Outside noises should be muffled so that they are distant and not distracting. The temperature must be comfortable, and the client and therapist must be able to relax.

For the client, the massage table should be comfortable, easy to climb onto, secure, and safe. Bolsters may be needed to ensure comfort, and the client must be warm.

For the therapist, body mechanics are essential. For long sessions on small areas of the body, like the face and neck, it is recommended that the therapist sit rather than stand. The height of the chair should be such that when the therapist sits back on the chair seat with the spine fully supported, the arms will rest comfortably on the table.

THE MEDITATIVE TOUCH

Lymph drainage massage is slow, light, repetitive, and rhythmical, and it requires the therapist to focus his or her attention very narrowly, counting the seconds and number of circles repetitively. To detect subtle changes in the soft tissue, the therapist must ignore distractions and focus attention only on the client. These subtle changes indicate that lymph fluid is moving in response to the work. With practice, the therapist can learn to maintain the appropriate level of touch, accompanied by perfectly smooth and rhythmical repetitions of the massage movements. As skill develops, the therapist can also learn to control his or her own breathing so that the repetitive cycle of massage movements harmonizes with the therapist's breath rate. The therapist can, for instance, practice inhaling slowly at the start of each circle and exhaling while releasing pressure and completing the massage circle. Eventually, this will become quite comfortable for the therapist, and he or she will be breathing at a rate that is conducive to meditation.

Such narrow focus, along with repetitive counting and relaxed breathing, will often put the therapist in a meditative state. Slow, repetitive massage movements, blending with the natural rhythms of the body, induce the same meditative state in the client. In this state, therapist and client can create an energetic bond. While stimulating lymph flow on a physiological level, LDM will relax the client's breath and heart rate, resulting in a balancing and harmonizing of the client's energy. This may explain why clients often report positive therapy outcomes that are not explained by the physiologic realities of the body and the massage. Apparently, inner work is also done.

For example, clients may drift off and, in dreamlike states, begin to review their lives in their minds, reframing incidents and understanding themes that alter their perspectives. In this state, the clients may also experience visions, flashbacks, or regressive experiences. They may feel unpleasant familiar or unfamiliar emotions, and they might have such physical symptoms such as pain from an old injury.

PREPARING THE CLIENT

Obviously, such inner experiences may be more than clients expect from massage. Although such experiences are beneficial, they are unsought and therefore may be unnerving. It is important, therefore, that therapists review the following guidelines.

Clients can relax more completely when they trust their therapists. Trust builds as clients sense congruity in their therapists and feel that their therapists have integrity. A client's sense of congruity in a therapist depends on the client seeing or sensing that the therapist practices what he or she believes, and is on a life path leading toward wholeness. Clients must feel sure that the therapist will never betray them or abuse their trust.

The therapist should recognize that the massage experience belongs to the client, not the therapist. The therapist should not take emotional outbursts personally, nor become involved. For example, the therapist should offer no advice about the client's personal experiences or problems.

If the client is distressed and upset, the therapist should remain calm and reassuring and offer a tissue if there are any tears. Sometimes, the relaxed dreamlike state is so real that clients are unsure where they are or what is happening. If this happens, the therapist should reassure the client and let the client know that he or she is safe.

Allow clients to explore the meanings of their inner experiences. Do not interpret. Instead, turn the clients back to their histories for understanding. It can be very tempting to try to explain an experience to a client, but it does not help, because it short-circuits their growth. Like dreams, a client's inner experiences during a body-mind session often contain universally recognized symbols. However, the symbol's real meaning for the client will be very individual. For instance, some clients may interpret the sensation of weightlessness as flying and they will feel free and exhilarated; others may interpret weightlessness as being disconnected and unstable, and possibly frightening. Rather than attempting to explain the experience, let the client know that many people have similar experiences in similar settings.

Do not invalidate an experience for a client by withdrawing or disapproving. This may be difficult if, say, the client experiences a past life and the therapist does not believe in past lives. Stay detached, focus on the LDM, and allow the client to realize the internal experience fully. If the client relates an extreme experience, such as an out-of-body experience or an alien abduction, the therapist should remain neutral and uninvolved. The therapist's job is to massage, not to counsel clients about their inner experiences. If the client wants the therapist to respond to his or her experience, the therapist should say that they lack the understanding or skills to deal with the experience. The therapist should then refer the client to someone who is qualified to discuss the matter.

It is important that therapists stay in touch with their own processes and reactions to clients' experiences. Client memories, emotions, and experiences can trigger possibly uncomfortable reactions in therapists, especially if the experiences have been the same for both client and therapist. Therapists may empathize, but they must keep their feelings separate from clients' feelings. The session must focus on the client. If the client has experiences that bring up uncomfortable memories for the therapist, the therapist should not discuss those feelings with the client. The therapist should seek counseling at another time, with another therapist.

Make sure clients are oriented and can drive safely before they leave. If clients have entered a meditative state, they will need time to return to full alertness. Physical reactions may be slower than usual, and clients may not be entirely aware of everything in their environment when leaving the table. Offer water, check their clothes to ensure they have buttoned things correctly, and stay with them until they are fully alert and able to drive safely.

One of the results of this kind of meditative work is that therapists, as well as clients, will experience meditative effects. Therapists who regularly perform meditative massage techniques may experience increased intuitive response to situations, periodic flashes of childhood trauma, turning away from some of the coarser demands of life, offending significant others by one's growth and change, desiring dietary changes, and so on. Therapists who are not ready for the life changes resulting from meditative practice may find themselves resistant to the discipline demanded by this kind of work: the slow, measured pace, and the focus and mindfulness necessary for effective therapy. Simple breathing exercises, as well as learning how to relax and slow down, will help.

Like their clients, estheticians or massage therapists may feel they are getting more than they bargained for when clients react to the work on many levels. When therapists are unprepared for this possibility, it can be overwhelming. The following information from Robert Leichtman, M.D., may help therapists to understand the reciprocal energetic effect of meditative body work. In a letter to Judy Dean, quoted with permission, Dr. Leichtman gave the following explanation of the energetic exchange that occurs in massage:

> "There are other even more subtle things going on when there is a therapeutic interaction between the client and the caregiver (of any type). Depending (a great amount) on the consciousness of the healer, the client is drawn into the aura (energy field) of the healer (person doing the massage, etc.). This is akin to a mother holding an infant, bathing the child in her affection and expectations. This sort of energetic radiation fills the energy field of the child or client. Usually, this will be a healthy experience unless, that is, that the person doing the treatment is full of conflict, anxiety or some other dark mood....
>
> "Now if the healer is in a higher, meditative state of mind, this higher level of awareness is also transmitted to the client. That is, just as a mother can draw a fussing infant into her maternal peace and quiet love of life, thereby soothing the infant, so also a healer can draw the client into a more

tranquil, meditative, contemplative state of mind. This can be a state of mind in which they can begin to register subtle insights and experience the state of goodwill, in which forgiveness, tolerance and letting go, can occur.

"As you undoubtedly know, the person who is loaded down with lots of unresolved conflict and gobs of retained fear, anger, doubt, guilt, grief, etc., will just retain it forever. The more tense, angry, full of self-pity, etc., we are, the more we keep the lid on these dark moods as well as add to them by the tendency to nurse grievances. They are released only as we cultivate a deeply relaxed state in which we can float in a quiet, contemplative state where the far more subtle healing forces of goodwill, self-respect, and wisdom can function. These are the healing states in which we can let go of anger, fear, guilt, and can allow healing insights to come to us.

"My point is, the higher state of wisdom, love, joy, and inclusive acceptance of the healer becomes a catalyst and stimulus for the client to reach a similar state. It is not just relaxation (or lymph flow). This higher state of consciousness is where psychological healing (as well as physical healing) can occur."[1]

HEALING CRISIS

Although the concept of a healing crisis is generally not recognized outside alternative therapies, massage therapists and others in similar fields have experienced this phenomenon in their practices. Clients who begin health regimens that depart from their customary lifestyles may experience difficult periods. They may re-experience symptoms of previous illnesses, such as childhood asthma. They may report that they taste antibiotics, although they have taken none in years. They may start to ache in the area of an old injury. These experiences are temporary, but they can be alarming if the therapist does not prepare the client for the experience.

A healing crisis can happen to clients who are receiving one or a series of lymph drainage massage sessions. Therapists should tell clients that occasionally people experience a slight malaise, flu symptoms or other symptoms, after massage. Instruct clients to drink fluids, rest, and in general, treat themselves as if they have the flu. A healing crisis is temporary and is accepted among alternative practitioners as a sign that therapy is working. If the symptoms last longer than three days, the client may actually be ill and should seek treatment.

Understanding the Health Crisis

The healing crisis is a purely non-medical empirical concept. The idea of the healing crisis is one of the underlying principles unique to alternative therapies that sets those therapies apart from mainstream medical practice. In practical terms, when a client begins to adopt a healthier lifestyle, he or she will sometimes feel worse before feeling better. Massage therapists and estheticians should be aware that their clients will sometimes experience healing crises following LDM. When they have been informed, clients generally feel positive about the experiences. Clients who have not been informed of the healing crisis can become alarmed and feel that massage work somehow harmed them. Therefore, communication is crucial, but it is also important not to overemphasize the possibility of a healing crisis, because it does not happen to everyone.

Start with educating the client about the lymphatic system. When clients understand that the lymphatic system does indeed remove toxins from the body, they will be less worried about transient symptoms related to toxin upheaval during or after the lymph massage. Explain that, since we live in a polluted world, the lymphatic system has a lot of work to do and that pollutants we inhale, ingest, or are exposed to in other ways may accumulate in the body. Lymph drainage massage stimulates the circulation of lymph and helps to remove toxins, and it's possible to feel a little worse before feeling better after the massage.

The concept of the healing crisis was developed in an attempt to explain the symptoms that clients report after massage and the observation of therapists that skilled touch readily activates both physical and nonphysical symptoms that can alarm the client. The truth is that lymph drainage massage affects the client on many levels beyond the lymphatic system. LDM affects the skin, muscles, the removal of metabolic waste, mood, pain, sleep and perhaps even the level of medication in the bloodstream. As time goes on, medical research will clarify our understanding of how LDM affects all these processes in the body. In the meantime, it is important to reassure clients that these symptoms sometimes happen and are mostly benign.

Healing crises are to be taken in stride. Generally, clients enjoy LDM and feel better, relaxed, and soothed afterward. A healing crisis will not occur with every client or with every massage session. When a healing crisis does occur, it can begin spontaneously during the LDM session or it can be precipitated by the work and occur later. The reaction may be physical (e.g., flu symptoms, shivering, mild nausea) or nonphysical (e.g., weeping, emotional release, visions). The healing crisis might involve releases on more than one level. For instance, the client may weep during the massage, remembering a childhood sorrow, then go home and suffer upper respiratory symptoms. When this kind of event occurs during a session, experienced practitioners realize that their responsibility is to remain with the client, quietly and sensitively, until the release is over.

With experience, practitioners will come to recognize clients who have greater potential for healing crises than others. Some clients are too fragile emotionally to weather the fallout of some treatments. Other clients may have simply neglected their health for so many years that a healing crisis is inevitable when they begin to change their lives, including the receiving of massage treatments. When in doubt, limit the length and frequency of lymph massage. Combine LDM with other massage techniques that have less potential for a healing crisis. Also, be prepared to refer clients to appropriate counselors or medical practitioners if they are having difficulty with memories or feelings experienced during or after the massage, or are feeling ill for more than three days after the session.

Dangers of Emotional Release Work

Clients who are experiencing emotional release can feel sad, angry, afraid, silly, libidinous, or child-like. The massage session may be further complicated if the client attempts to repress or hold in the emotional memories because he or she feels the emotions are unacceptable, for instance, if the client is experiencing fear or anger. The client may feel tremendously sad and not know why. The client may become sexually aroused and either act out inappropriately or feel shame and embarrassment, or the client may be afraid of ridicule or ostracism. This can be very confusing for the client and the therapist.

The therapist's job is to communicate, listen, and not become involved. First, assure the client that these feelings are normal; everyone has feelings trapped in muscles and when the muscles are massaged, the feelings release and arise. Assure the client that the feelings will go away, and that they are historical feelings. They are related to events in the past, not the present. If the client is very distressed, or is recovering repressed memories of seriously damaging events in the past, refer the client to an appropriate therapist. Do not attempt to counsel the client or rescue the client in any way. The therapist's job is to give the massage.

Learn to be present with the client without feeling that you have to solve the problem. Being present includes paying attention to what is said, adjusting or changing the work you are doing as necessary, providing tissues or water if needed, and reassuring the client that many people feel this way when they have been stressed for a long time. However, it is important to repeat that the massage therapist should not try to solve the client's problems.

The therapist can be just as confused as the client. The therapist may need to say this out loud and ask the client how he or she is feeling and what is happening. For instance, if the client seems to be angry and the therapist isn't sure why, it is better to ask what is happening. The client may be angry about any number of things, which may or may not have anything to do with the therapist. If the therapist is doing something the client doesn't like, the therapist will never know if he/she doesn't ask. If the anger is muscle memory, it will be helpful if the client can identify the memory that made him/her angry. A client's anger can be intimidating to the therapist, and the therapist may react in fear, further confusing the issue. Communication can diffuse the situation and provide clarity.

The client's experience can mesh with a previous experience of the therapist, which can also be confusing and can cause the therapist to act inappropriately. If the client has a history of having been abused, for instance, in a way that the therapist also has been abused, the therapist will identify with the client and may want to rescue him/her or be angry on his/her behalf. It is important for therapists to understand their own emotional triggers, and remain detached.

Respect the client's boundaries and avoid invasive or intrusive questions or comments. Making suggestions about how to solve the client's problems is invasive, as are personal comments, for instance about the client's appearance, dress, income, family or other personal matters. The therapist has a right to ask questions about a client's health history, medications, expectations for the massage and so on, but should avoid inappropriate questions or the giving of advice.

When a client makes personal revelations to the therapist while experiencing emotional release, the therapist could assume that there is a level of intimacy that doesn't really exist if there is a lack of boundaries, or lack of understanding. The therapist should at all times remain professional in his/her behavior and not attempt a more personal relationship with the client.

A massage therapist who isn't clear about his/her role can be tempted to create dependency in a client by attempting to solve the client's problems or rescue the client from his/her problems. Creating dependency in a client may stroke the therapist's ego but it also creates a burden the therapist will eventually resent. It also interferes with the client's growth and maturity. People grow and change best when they are allowed to solve their own problems.

Other Problems from Emotional Release Work: Interpretation

The massage therapist generally doesn't have enough information to interpret the client's experience and should not attempt to explain the memories or other experiences the client may have during massage. Allow the client to find the meaning in the experience.

Identification

Identification means imposing your issues on the client as an explanation of what the client is experiencing. Clients may sometimes express feelings or describe events that trigger memories in the therapist. However, the situations may not be the same at all. Be very careful about sharing personal experiences with clients, or about judging the client in terms of your own personal experiences. Remember that your experiences and feelings are separate from the client's experiences and feelings.

Enmeshment

It is easy for a sympathetic person to become inappropriately involved in the client's life and to establish a personal relationship instead of maintaining the business relationship. Therapists who find themselves helping clients outside of the massage room, running errands or giving them rides for instance, should re-evaluate their own boundaries.

Judgment

It is also easy for the therapist to judge the client by his/her own standards. The client is bad or good depending on how his/her experience seems to the therapist. For instance, a therapist may think a client who smokes is "bad" and "doesn't care about his health." It is important to stay detached and resist making judgments about our clients. Their lives are their own business and they don't have to answer to their massage therapists about how they live.

People-pleaser

You may believe that the client's feelings apply to something about you, and either become distressed because you think you aren't pleasing the client. Then you may allow the client to violate your boundaries out of your desire to please, giving longer sessions for no extra fee, for instance, or allowing the client to interfere with your personal life. You may feel that you can't say "no" to a client, or that you have to explain your decisions to your clients. You may find yourself frequently making changes that are inconvenient to you in order to accommodate your clients. If you don't enforce your own boundaries, you may begin to resent your clients because they take up too much time and energy.

Remember that if you can keep quiet, clients can do their own internal work. The massage therapist provides the setting and the bodywork, which give the client the space and opportunity to grow. Don't judge, interrupt, or interpret. Don't make suggestions or offer any help other than bodywork. Breathe and stay calm. Resist the temptation to do something about your client's emotional pain.

Boundaries

Be careful about how you comfort a person in distress. Remember that the client is naked, protected only by the drape and by the therapist's good intentions. The client is emotionally vulnerable. Maintain crisp boundaries and remain professional. Avoid the temptation to hug the client. A needy or distressed client could misinterpret hugging or other personal touch; it could even be offensive to some. It sends mixed messages about the therapist's role in the relationship.

Be aware of spiritual boundaries. Don't impose your spiritual path on your client. In fact, the client's spiritual beliefs are not the business of the therapist; they don't have to explain or justify their beliefs in order to get a massage.

You may feel the compulsion to fix the client or solve the client's problems, doing more than your job. For instance, this could include giving the client a ride somewhere, loaning money or doing a massage for free, or creating a social/personal relationship out of what ought to be a business relationship. You may crave a client's praise and continually set up situations where the client gives that praise. It helps to be self-aware, to have knowledge of your own weaknesses, so that you can set up and maintain absolutely crisp boundaries.

It is easier to maintain professional boundaries if you dress professionally, speak professionally, focus on the work at hand and avoid chatting with clients about personal matters.

REVIEW QUESTIONS

1. Explain the importance of the setting for the massage.
2. What elements of the massage produce a meditative state?
3. Why is it important to set boundaries in a massage? What boundaries could you set that help to protect your client?
4. What can occur when a client enters a relaxed dreamlike state during the massage?
5. What mistakes might you make with a client if you don't honor your own boundaries and your client's boundaries when the client is in a relaxed dreamlike state?

6. What subtle responses can happen during a lymph drainage massage that might surprise the client or the therapist?
7. What is a healing crisis? What causes it?
8. How should a therapist or esthetician handle a client's emotional release?
9. How would you handle it if your client becomes angry during a massage?
10. How would you handle it if your client begins to cry during a massage?

Using Lymph Drainage Massage with Other Treatments

L ymph drainage massage can be easily and effectively combined with other techniques, including:

- Sports massage, to speed the healing of injuries and reduce inflammation and edema
- Deep-tissue massage, to reduce post-session soreness and swelling
- Facials, to enhance the skin from the inside and outside
- Body-mind work, to produce a deeply relaxed state for inner work
- Detoxifying treatments, to speed the removal of cellular waste and stimulate the circulation and reproduction of immune cells
- Cellulite therapy, to speed the removal of toxins and reduce edema and inflammation

SOFT-TISSUE INJURY

Lymph drainage massage very effectively reduces swelling and speeds healing. The therapist must take precautions to avoid complicating an injury or acute condition. Consider the following information before performing lymph drainage massage on a person who has been injured recently, who is postoperative, or who is suffering acute pain and swelling.

Following an injury, and before any LDM is undertaken, the client must obtain medical attention to rule out broken bones, torn ligaments or muscles, and any other massage contraindications. Open wounds, surgeries, and the like must heal before tissues are touched by a massage therapist. Postsurgical massage work must not be undertaken until enough time has elapsed for healing in order to avoid contaminating the incision or wound, and to be sure that no blood clots have formed. The best way to ensure this is to insist on a prescription for LDM from the client's physician as long as the client is still under the physician's care. This request is usually honored, and the prescription signifies that the patient has been properly cleared for massage by a licensed medical professional. Once clients have been released by their physicians and need no more follow-up visits, massage may be assumed safe.

Infection, if any, must have healed, as it is a serious LDM contraindication.

When the client is ready for lymph drainage massage, use it to reduce swelling and speed healing. Follow the standard procedures for lymph drainage massage as described in other chapters in this text. Be aware that the greater the edema, the longer it will take to reduce. This requires more repetitions of the massage strokes, possibly as many as 100 repetitions in each area.

Massage the appropriate lymph nodes first, and the tissue between the lymph nodes and the injury. Work around the perimeter of the swelling or injury, gradually working into the center of the injury. Work toward the center of the injury slowly, within the patient's or client's tolerance, as the area may be painful. Finish by massaging from the injury or incision back to the lymph nodes again, moving fluid toward the lymph nodes. Massage the lymph nodes again. If there is a great deal of swelling in the injured area, the therapist may have to work back and forth between the nodes and the injury several times in a session to keep the nodes and proximal tissue clear.

When the preceding precautions have been observed, LDM may be safely performed daily. When progress is maintained for 24 hours, give sessions every other day or every third day. As the condition improves, gradually lengthen the time between sessions. If the client cannot have daily sessions, instruct the client to self-treat.

REDUCING FIBROSIS AND SCAR TISSUE

When an injury or a surgery has healed, the client's readiness for other work can be assessed by considering whether the client reports that the pain has decreased or disappeared, the wound or surgery has obviously healed and swelling has reduced, and no infection (local or general) is present.

The next step is to reduce muscle contracture, fibrosis and scar tissue. Following that, muscles must be retrained to balance movement.

Deep-tissue massage may be used to relieve muscle contracture, break down fibroids, break down or prevent adhesions, and reduce scar tissue. Deep tissue massage refers to massage that focuses on connective tissue, working slowly through muscle layers until all the muscles are relaxed. Deep tissue massage does NOT mean using forceful pressure to reach deeper muscles. Like LDM, deep tissue massage is a subtle technique. It must be used with care to avoid damaging the client. Deep massage work performed hastily and with too much force can damage lymph capillaries, even in a healthy person.

There can be a buildup of **fibrotic** tissue in and around a previously injured area, due to the inflammation that occurred. This makes the muscles and skin coarser, less flexible, and colder than normal. Deep-tissue massage (connective tissue massage) can be used to break down fibrosis and make muscles and skin smoother, more flexible, and warmer. Deep tissue massage also breaks down and even prevents adhesions.

Use friction strokes across and along the length of scars and keloid ridges. It is safe to massage scars daily, stretching the scar tissue until a slight burning sensation is felt in the scar. Because one side effect of deep-tissue massage is inflammation, follow deep-tissue activities with LDM in order to reduce inflammation and prevent additional swelling.

As the client heals and tissue returns to normal, encourage the client to do stretching exercises to maintain progress. Engage the client in the healing process by encouraging home follow-up. In injury rehabilitation work, it is important to guide the client in stretching exercises that relax and retrain affected muscles. Strengthening exercises may also be needed, as muscles may have become weak while healing.

Encourage clients to undergo movement training to prevent new injuries and to restore muscle balance. For example, clients who are athletes should have some training from a coach. Others, like those learning yoga or tai chi, benefit from movement training as a way to increase wellness. Encourage clients to participate in these activities.

LDM can be used effectively with deep-tissue massage even when there is no edema or scar tissue. LDM reduces post-session soreness and swelling. Deep-tissue massage focuses on connective tissue, using specific strokes to change posture and movement, and reduce scar tissue and chronic muscle contracture.

Deep-tissue massage movements elongate and relax muscles by creating microtears in the connective tissue of the muscle. It is often combined with stretching or other movement training to ensure that the muscle remains relaxed and stretched while healing. Deep-tissue massage produces inflammation as a side effect. Following deep-tissue massage with LDM reduces inflammation, speeds healing of microtears, and helps new scar tissue in the muscle form correctly.

COMPLEMENTING SKIN CARE

LDM is used in the beauty industry as an important part of skin care. LDM improves the skin's appearance and texture, reducing the fibrosis and damage resulting from exposure to cold and sun. LDM also improves circulation, bringing in nutrition for skin cells, and removing cellular waste and disease-causing microorganisms.

BODY-MIND THERAPIES

LDM is ideal for body-mind therapies because it is gentle, extremely relaxing, and, in the right circumstances, trance inducing. The very slow pace and regular rhythm of lymph drainage massage help to induce a meditative state of consciousness in which clients can do internal work. Combining breathwork with LDM assists in producing a meditative state in the client. More skilled therapists can modulate their breathing with their own pulse rate, producing a fundamental rhythm that then enhances the massage work for the client.

DETOXIFICATION TREATMENTS

Spas and massage clinics offer a wide variety of body treatments such as scrubs, wraps, and applications of seaweed, clays, mud, and herbal preparations. There is no doubt that body treatments are a wonderful experience, but the spa industry also claims that there are health benefits. These claims are often based on tradition, and the most common claim is that the body treatments remove "toxins" from the body, without identifying exactly what those toxins are.

Body wraps are an ancient tool used to combat disease. European and American spas and sanatoria of the 19th century used combinations of massage, body wraps, sweats, and hydrotherapy to help their chronically ill patients regain health. Since ancient times, northern cultures have used what scientists call "whole body hyperthermia" to maintain health and cure disease, in the form of saunas, sweat lodges, and body wraps. When Queen Elizabeth I had smallpox, she was wrapped closely in sheets with only her head and one hand exposed until her fever broke and she began to sweat, and eventually recovered from the illness.

There is a scientific basis for using lymph drainage massage, body wraps and other spa services for reasons of health. Studies show that whole body hyperthermia, or an artificial fever, increases the activity, mobility, and reproduction of white blood cells, our primary defense against disease on a cellular level.

In one study, scientists subjected mice to whole body hyperthermia, somewhat akin to putting the mice in a dry sauna, to determine the effect of fever on the production and activities of white blood cells. The study showed that there is an increase in white blood cell activity when the body's core temperature is raised.[1,2]

In another study on fish, gradually raising the temperature of the water around the fish reduced the occurrence and virulence of infections because of increased immune activity in the fish. This explained why the rate of infections in wild fish goes down in the springtime as water temperatures go up.[3,4,5]

In fact, the use of externally applied hyperthermia in cancer therapies has been shown to increase the mobility and activity of white blood cells in tumors.[6,7,8,9,10]

However, if a temperature is used that is higher than a natural fever, even if immune activities in the cells are supported, it can be damaging. Using temperatures within the natural fever range has been found to produce little damage while maintaining the benefits of a natural fever.[11]

As far as massage goes, the January 2005 Mayo Clinic Health Letter reports that massage improves circulation, improves blood pressure, and relieves fluid buildup in the arms and legs. According to the newsletter, massage releases stress-reducing hormones, reduces pain, anxiety, stress and depression, improves the range of motion, and helps with many conditions including arthritis, lymphedema disease, and fibromyalgia. The Touch Research Institute reports that massage therapy improves immune function.[12]

So the bottom line is that body wraps, combined with lymph drainage massage, can and do stimulate the activities of the immune system, enhancing health and resistance to disease.

Does a body wrap used with lymph drainage massage remove toxins from the body? Toxins are microorganisms, microscopic particles, and chemicals that are harmful to the organism. The body responds by sending white blood cells to attack the invading microorganisms or other toxins. So massage and spa treatments that increase the mobility, activity and reproduction of white blood cells do help to remove toxins from the body by stimulating natural processes.

Are there any contraindications to "whole body hyperthermia" whether in a body wrap, sauna, or hot tub? These treatments are not recommended for anyone with uncontrolled high blood pressure or for anyone who is pregnant. Also, body wraps are not recommended for anyone with severe claustrophobia, although for mild claustrophobia, the therapist can arrange the wrap so that, like Queen Elizabeth I, one arm is outside the wrap. Also, it is important for the client to be well-hydrated, which means having a drink of water before beginning the treatment, and having water available during the session.

Therapists should be aware that combining therapies, such as wraps or fasting, with LDM can trigger a healing crisis. The combination can make the client feel ill with flulike symptoms, for example. Body wraps work by creating an artificial fever, increasing body heat, and have the same effects on the body as a genuine fever in response to pathogens. If the therapist feels that a client may react to the combination of treatments with a healing crisis, it is better not to combine the therapies, but to offer the treatments as separate sessions on different days. If a client is responding to fasting with symptoms of illness, wait to offer LDM until the client is no longer fasting. It will still be effective in helping the immune system to remove cellular waste and disease-causing organisms. To be sure that internal body temperature does not exceed safe limits during a body wrap, the client's temperature should be taken and should not exceed 100 degrees Fahrenheit.

CELLULITE

Cellulite is a controversial subject. It does or does not exist according to whom one consults. Although medical practitioners do not acknowledge cellulite's existence by and large, practitioners in the massage, beauty, and skin care industries think it is real, treat it as if it were real, and achieve positive outcomes.

Introducing Cellulite

Cellulite is an unscientific, descriptive term. It was first used in Sweden at the end of the nineteenth century and was adopted by French salons to refer to the dimpled, rippling appearance of the skin, usually over the buttocks, thighs, and abdomen.

It is sometimes called lipedema, although that is an inaccurate use of the term. Cellulite refers to the appearance of the skin. Lipedema refers to the proliferation of fat cells in chronically edematous tissue.

Cellulite most commonly appears on the hips, the thighs, and the upper arms. On older women, it may also appear across the upper back, across the abdomen, and even on the calves. To the touch, the texture of cellulite is lumpy and discontinuous, and when squeezed or palpated, cellulite appears as lumps and masses. The appearance of cellulite is unfortunate at the least, and positively disfiguring in severe cases. The tendency toward cellulite can be inherited, although lifestyle and diet play a major role in its formation.

Cellulite should be differentiated from obesity. In cellulite, fat cells may be normal, but the connective tissue is damaged, which contributes to the rippled and lumpy appearance of the skin. Cellulite is distributed mainly in the well-known "saddlebag" area, over the hips, abdomen, and thighs, in non-obese women. Other areas of the body are normal in size and appearance. Cellulite has two components: an unattractive distribution of fat cells below the waist and a disturbance of the connective tissue, which causes scarring and distortion of the superficial fascia. Cellulite can also include true edema, which is an abnormal accumulation of fluid in these regions. Manual massage therapies are effective in treating the scarring of the connective tissue and the edema, but cannot remove or redistribute fat cells.

Obesity is not due to a proliferation of fat cells, but an increase in the size of fat cells due to taking in too much energy in the form of food. It is not located only in the saddlebag area below the waist, but is distributed over the entire body. LDM cannot reduce the amount or size of fat stored in the body. However, over time, the seriously obese patient will develop edema in the lower extremities, marked by pitting edema and pathological changes to the skin. Because chronic edema can develop into more serious conditions, such as chronic infections or even some forms of cancer, it is important to treat the edema. The condition cannot be successfully cured unless the obesity is also addressed.

Cellulite forms in the superficial fascia, a layer of connective tissue below the skin that contains fat cells. The superficial fascia is fibrous and, due to inactivity, injuries, and improper exercise, adhesions (scar tissue) in the fascia can form, contributing to the bunched-up or rippled look of the skin. Not only does the superficial fascia become more fibrous, thickened, coarse, and less flexible, but it can also adhere to underlying structures that it normally slides over.

Improper exercise is also a factor in cellulite. Lack of exercise causes one set of problems, including weak muscles, poor skin tone, sluggish lymph circulation, and weight gain. Overexercise causes another set of problems: tense, overworked muscles contributing to fatigue and the buildup of the by-products of the combustion of energy. Overworked, fatigued muscles are easily injured, leading to tears in the connective tissue that, in turn, lead to the development of scar tissue and adhesions. Excessive exercise combined with very strict dieting can lead to malnutrition, which adversely affects the appearance and texture of the skin.

Obesity, sun, gravity, and exposure to cold can cause changes in the skin, ranging from atrophy to hypertrophy. If the collagen of the skin is damaged, changes take place such as accumulation of fat cells and thickened skin. Fat cells can change in size, depending on exercise and diet. All of these conditions contribute to the appearance of cellulite.

Remedying Cellulite

The ultimate remedy is to enhance the body's circulation, improve nutrition, increase metabolism, and reduce scar tissue and adhesions in the superficial fascia. Treatment of cellulite requires more than just LDM. A successful program has to include changes in diet and lifestyle.

Treating the Body

The most effective bodywork treatment of cellulite combines connective tissue massage, or myofascial release, to break down adhesions in the superficial tissues and increase nutrition to the tissues, with gentle lymphatic massage to remove inflammation and toxins.

Deep tissue massage and myofascial release focus on connective tissue. The deep, slow massage strokes produce their effect by creating microtears in the superficial fascia. This makes tissue longer, smoother, and more flexible. The deep massage work also releases adhesions in the superficial fascia so that tissue moves more freely and no longer adheres to underlying structures. Deep massage followed by LDM and appropriate stretching make the superficial fascia smoother, longer, and more flexible, improving the appearance of the skin.

Creating tears in the superficial fascia with deep-tissue massage or myofascial release triggers the inflammatory response. Blood flow increases and capillaries become more permeable, thereby increasing nutrition to the tissues. Increased blood flow increases the amount of interstitial fluid, which in turn washes the cells and picks up microorganisms and foreign particles. LDM stimulates the removal of these toxins through the lymphatic system.

In this context, it is important to note that although superficial lymphatic capillaries are connected to deeper vessels via pathways through the adipose (fatty) tissue, they provide very little effective drainage of the fat cells. It is inaccurate to let clients believe that massage will remove or decrease fat cells. What bodywork *will* do is greatly improve the condition and appearance of the skin, reduce troublesome adhesions and scars, and increase the circulation of nutrients to tissues. As a result of the bodywork, the body will repair itself and move to a higher level of health and appearance.

The most successful treatment that actually removes fat cells from the body and restructures the shape of the body is liposuction. The surgical removal of fat cells can be used to reshape saddlebags on the hips, the rear end, abdomen, and any other area of the body where fat cells have accumulated, such as under the chin. However, the procedure itself damages the connective tissue, blood vessels, and lymph vessels in the area of the surgery. This can create more scarring if the procedure is not performed skillfully and if there is no follow-up. Scarring due to liposuction can cause edema, and chronic edema can lead to a worsening of the appearance of the skin, rather than improvement.

Clients who want to have liposuction should research carefully and select physicians who are experienced, and who have a history of obtaining good results. It is important to select a physician who is interested not only in doing the surgery, but also in educating the client to obtain the best possible result.

Once the surgery has healed, LDM is recommended because it can help the proper development of scar tissue, improve circulation, and assist in the removal of damaged tissues and chemicals. Deep-tissue massage is not recommended until the area has completely healed and there is no tenderness.

Cellulite responds well to regular connective tissue massage or myofascial release, and LDM. Note that deep massage techniques should not be applied to the same area of the body more than once every third day. LDM, however, may be given daily. Encourage clients to commit to a series of bodywork sessions, such as six in two weeks, for cellulite work. Then suggest less frequent bodywork sessions while the client works on changing diet and implementing an exercise program to maintain the progress achieved by the bodywork.

OUTLINE OF CELLULITE MASSAGE

Gather materials: oil or cream, bolster for knees, small roll to place under the neck, small blanket or towel for warmth. For connective tissue massage, use little or no lubricant. Choose lotion that is quickly absorbed or an oil (like coconut oil) that is thin and has more drag than glide. Use sparingly. Cellulite creams such as those containing arnica and ivy may be applied at the end of the session.

Before beginning the session, ask the client to stand, wearing only underwear or a bathing suit. Examine the cellulite. Observe the contour of the hips and legs, the texture and condition of the skin, and any markings including scar tissue, moles, lumps, etc. To measure progress, the therapist may want to measure the circumference of the hips and thighs, marking the level where the measurement is taken with a nontoxic, waxy pencil such as eyeliner. To record the measurement, measure the distance from a landmark such as the knee crease (e.g., seven inches above the posterior knee crease) and note any changes in circumference at that point.

The therapist may also wish to take pictures of the area to be worked. However, photos should not be taken without prior permission from the client, and at the end of the treatment period, the photographs should be returned to the client.

Explain the procedure to the client, so there are no surprises or unanswered questions. Assist the client onto the massage table, in a prone position. Drape warmly, and uncover the area to be massaged.

Assess the condition of the skin: color, texture, temperature, moisture, and elasticity. Look at the contour of the hips and legs. Look for skin thickening, ridges, lumps, and wrinkles. Examine visible scars for any that will run across lymph vessels, because these will obstruct lymph drainage. Look for pockets of edema and feel the tissues around the edematous areas, palpating for thickness, stiff tissue, or fibrotic tissue. Examine visible veins, looking for redness, swelling, heat, and pain. To assist in remembering the appearance of the skin before cellulite treatment, make notes on an outline of the figure, marking the location of scars, edema, moles, veins, and so on, and describing them.

Connective Tissue Massage

Begin the connective tissue massage. Skin rolling is a good technique to reduce adhesions in the superficial fascia, the layer holding the fat cells. Pick up the skin between the thumb and fingers. Roll it over the thumb in a continuous motion, beginning at the gluteal crease and working toward the waist. The fingers walk along, picking up tissue, and the thumbs follow, pushing through the tissue. Cover the entire gluteal region with skin rolling. Then use skin rolling on the posterior thighs, rolling from the knee to the gluteal crease. Repeat until the entire area is covered and the skin is flushed and warm. The purpose of this initial movement is to release the superficial fascia from underlying structures and improve its flexibility.

The purpose of the next stroke is to create a mesh of microtears in the superficial fascia, which will stretch and smooth the fascia. Press down into the skin with the tips of the fingers, the flat hand, a flat fist, or the lower arm in front of the elbow. Press into the skin very slowly until resistance is met. At that level, begin sliding very slowly from the gluteal crease to the waist. Use lighter pressure over bony regions such as the iliac crest (the bony protuberance at the waist in the back). Repeat until the tissue in this area is warm, soft, and very pliable. The client should experience a light burning sensation, but no intense pain. If the work is painful, use less pressure and move even more slowly.

Repeat the deep stroke on the posterior thighs, from the knee to the gluteal crease. Use lighter pressure over the soft area behind the knee, and deeper pressure up the back of the thigh to the hip joint. Repeat until the entire posterior thigh on both legs have been worked.

Apply a cellulite cream if desired to the buttocks and thighs. Assist the client to turn over to a supine position. Drape warmly, but expose the hips and thighs. Use skin rolling if possible on the anterior thigh. Some clients will not be able to tolerate it. Follow with a deep stroke from above the knee to the inguinal ligament. Use lighter pressure over the medial thigh. *Do not* perform the deep massage stroke over the femoral triangle where the lymph nodes and femoral nerve and artery are located. Repeat the deep massage stroke over the entire anterior thigh (except as cautioned above) until the thigh is warm, flushed, and supple.

Lymph Drainage Massage

Begin LDM with the client in the supine position on the massage table. Massage the inguinal lymph nodes with very slow, stationary circles, using light pressure, for two to three minutes. Each circle should last seven seconds.

Massage the abdomen in a fan-shaped pattern. Place hands over the abdomen between the inguinal ligament and the navel, with the fingertips along the body's midline and the heels of the hands near the inguinal ligament. Using both hands, move the skin of the abdomen in large slow circles, with seven circles lasting seven seconds each, for about one minute.

Move hands so that the fingertips are along the waist, with the heels of the hands being close to the inguinal ligament, and massage as before for one minute.

Move hands so that the fingertips reach down the side of the body close to the massage table, between the waist and hip joint, with the heels of the hands near the inguinal ligament as before. Massage with slow circles, seven seconds per circle, for one minute.

If necessary, repeat the abdominal massage until there is a palpable change in the tissue.

Massage along the "side seam" of the thigh. Place hands over the upper third of the iliotibial band, near the hip joint, and massage using slow, stationary circles for about one minute. Each circle should take seven seconds, nearly one minute altogether.

Place hands over the middle third of the iliotibial band, and massage using slow, stationary circles. Each circle should take seven seconds, nearly one minute altogether.

Place hands over the lower third of the iliotibial band, near the knee, and massage using slow, stationary circles. Each circle should take seven seconds, nearly one minute altogether.

Place hands over the upper third of the thigh, inferior to the inguinal crease, covering the upper rectus femoris muscle, and massage using slow, stationary circles. Repeat circles seven times.

Place hands over the middle rectus femoris muscle area, and massage using stationary circles. Repeat circles seven times.

Place hands over the bottom of the rectus femoris muscle, superior to the knee, and massage using stationary circles. Repeat circles seven times.

Roll the knee out slightly, away from the midline, to make access to the inner thigh easier. Place hands over the lower half of the medial thigh and massage using stationary circles. Repeat circles seven times.

Place hands around the knee and use a scooping motion to move fluid toward the inguinal lymph nodes. Each "scoop" should take seven seconds, and should be repeated seven times. (A scoop is a semicircle.) Place one hand on each side of the knee, compress slightly, and stretch the skin in a semicircle toward the inguinal lymph nodes. Then release the pressure and return to the point of origin.

Repeat the LDM strokes in reverse order, working from the knee to the inguinal crease.

Massage the inguinal nodes for two to three minutes.

Assist the client into a prone position on the massage table. Using flat hands, massage the gluteal region in a fan-shaped pattern. Place hands so that the heels of the hands are close to the hip joint with fingers parallel to the gluteal crease. Massage using slow circles (each circle should last seven seconds). Repeat seven times.

Place hands so that the heels of the hands are close to the hip joint with fingers pointing toward the sacrum, and massage for one minute, using slow, stationary circles, seven seconds each circle.

Place the hands so that the heels of the hands are close to the hip joint with fingers pointing toward the waist, parallel to the massage table. Massage for one minute as before.

Massage the lumbar region, using stationary circles repeated seven times.

Massage over the sacrum using stationary circles.

Massage over the back of the knee to open the popliteal nodes using stationary circles. Repeat seven times.

Place flat hands on the upper thigh, just below the gluteal crease. Massage for one minute with stationary circles. Repeat seven times.

Place flat hands mid-thigh, with the fingers of each hand reaching down to the massage table on each side. Massage for one minute, moving the skin in a semicircle up toward the inguinal crease and out to the sides of the thigh. Repeat seven times, each scooping movement lasting about seven seconds.

Place flat hands just above the knee on the lower thigh, with fingers reaching to the massage table on each side. Move the skin in a semicircle up toward the inguinal crease and out to the sides of the thigh, repeating the scooping movement seven times, seven seconds each time.

Massage the back of the knee, using stationary circles for one minute. Each circle should last seven seconds.

Assist client to turn over into the supine position. Drape warmly. Finish the lower quadrant by massaging over the inguinal nodes again, twenty circles.

The cellulite treatment can be followed with a body wrap. Remember that the total session, including deep tissue massage, LDM and body wrap, should not exceed an hour and a half. The body wrap is not recommended for anyone who is pregnant or who has high blood pressure.

At the end of the session, encourage the client to stretch daily, drink water, and eat fruits and vegetables.

Self-Massage Using Lymph Drainage Massage Techniques

Nurses, estheticians, massage therapists, and other similar caregivers are as much educators as they are therapists and technicians. Teaching clients to understand the purpose and effects of the therapy is always beneficial and encourages compliance. This is especially true with LDM. Teaching one's clients to self-treat is valuable for several reasons. First, many clients cannot afford daily LDM sessions, but progress is more significant with daily therapy. Teaching clients to self-treat daily with weekly professional sessions yields better results than if the clients simply come in once a week for LDM sessions with professionals.

Besides self-treatment for lymphedema, clients may want to perform self-massage for beauty and health reasons. Daily lymph massage of the face and neck helps to maintain the skin in the best possible condition. Massaging the tissues of the face and neck, especially the lymph nodes, when the client feels a cold or another minor illness coming on helps to stimulate lymph circulation and the circulation of immune cells in the lymph vessels and nodes. Clients who suffer chronic sinus infections and nasal allergies will find LDM of the face very comforting.

People whose work demands that they stand all day, and who suffer edema and painful legs and feet as a result, will find that daily LDM helps to reduce edema, improve circulation, and reduce or eliminate leg pain. Obese patients who suffer from edema, especially in the lower extremities, will find that daily self-massage reduces the edema, improves circulation, reduces pain, and helps to prevent pathological changes to the skin that are common in chronic edema.

Women who suffer hormone-related bloating, and breast swelling and tenderness will find that regular LDM helps to eliminate each of these symptoms. Daily breast massage is important for breast health. Besides increasing lymph circulation and keeping breast tissues healthy, women who massage their breasts regularly will become very familiar with the way their breasts feel and will be able to detect subtle changes in breast tissue more quickly than with monthly breast self-examinations.

Knowing LDM basics enables family members to help each other with pain, edema, and scar tissue following soft-tissue injuries. Many painful soft-tissue problems, such as muscle tension, muscle spasm, inflammation, and overuse injuries, respond to LDM.

Teamwork on the part of the therapist or esthetician and the client produces the best results. It is a good idea to teach clients to self-treat so they can continue treatment between appointments with professional therapists. Routine self-massage helps to maintain the progress obtained in the professional session and allows the therapist to make greater progress during each session.

It is important for clients to understand the contraindications and appropriate use of LDM. When teaching clients simple techniques for self-massage, therapists should also make sure that clients understand when *not* to perform LDM.

Therapists can demonstrate simple procedures and help clients practice movements, and then in the next session discuss the client's experience with self-massage and refine the client's skill.

SELF-MASSAGING THE FACE AND NECK

Self-massage of the face and neck can be performed while sitting or lying. Probably the best position is seated with the back, neck, and head supported. The client is less likely to fall asleep if seated while practicing self-massage.

The basic principles for self-massage are the same as for professional massage therapists and estheticians. Using light pressure (1/2 to 8 ounces per square inch), move the skin in a circular or semicircular direction, repeating the moves regularly and slowly, six to ten repetitions a minute, and move lymph toward the lymph nodes.

Because the massage of the head and neck takes half an hour or more, some might find it easier to do the massage in sections, massaging the neck one day and the face the next. The work can be done with or without lotion or cream; it is a matter of preference. Heat stimulates lymph circulation, so steaming the face and neck first with a hot, moist towel is a good idea. Allow the moist, hot towel to cool to room temperature while massaging the face lightly through the towel.

Focusing on the Neck

STEP-BY-STEP

Seated comfortably, begin with the lymph nodes. Place the hands above the clavicle, next to the sternocleidomastoid muscles. Massage this area for two to three minutes using stationary circles, about seven per minute. It helps to have a loudly ticking clock nearby to count the seconds to make sure the massage movements are consistent. Stationary circles should last six to ten seconds, which is very slow. The natural tendency is to move faster unless one is watching a clock.

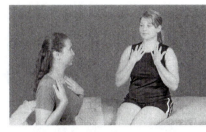

Massage the cervical nodes. Place flat fingers over the sternocleidomastoid muscles on either side of the neck, spreading the fingers to cover the muscles from the ear to the medial ends of the clavicle at the bottom of the throat. Massage lightly for at least one minute. Then, place flat fingers on the sides of the neck between the ear and the top of the shoulder, and massage lightly for another minute, about seven circles.

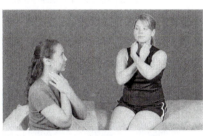

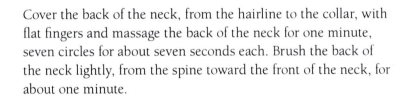

Cover the back of the neck, from the hairline to the collar, with flat fingers and massage the back of the neck for one minute, seven circles for about seven seconds each. Brush the back of the neck lightly, from the spine toward the front of the neck, for about one minute.

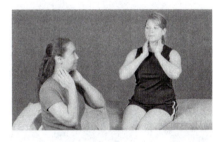

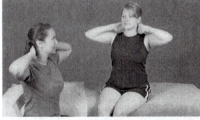

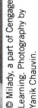

Massage the front of the neck gently, for about a minute. Brush the front of the neck lightly from the midline back to the sternocleidomastoid muscles.

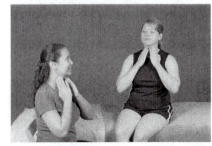

STEP-BY-STEP   Massaging the Face

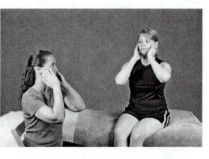

Massage the ring of lymph nodes under the jawline and the occiput. First, massage the pre- and post-auricular nodes.

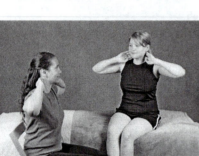

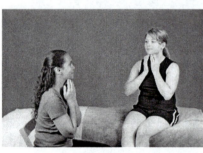

Next, massage the submandibular and submental nodes.

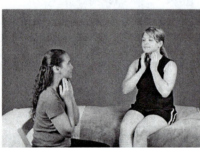

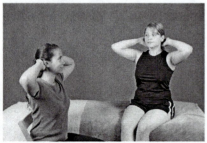

Massage the suboccipital nodes.

Massage the chin with flat fingertips for about one minute. Use seven circles per minute, watching a clock to maintain consistent speed.

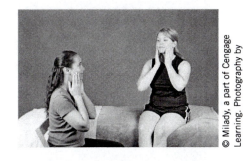
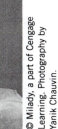

Then, using all fingertips, massage just above the jawline, from the corners of the mouth to the angle of the jaw, for about one minute.

Place flat fingers and the palm over the angle of the jaw, covering the area of the molars.

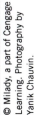

Then, massage the upper lip using one or two fingers of each hand, for about one minute.

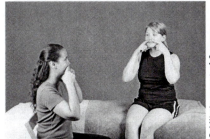

Use one or two fingers of each hand to massage the nose for one minute, about seven circles.

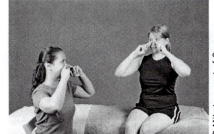

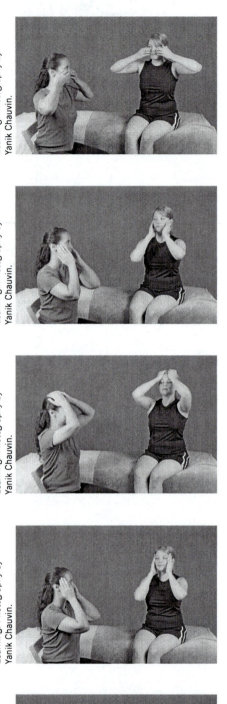

Place fingertips in the curve that runs from the inner corners of the eye to the corners of the mouth. Massage for at least one minute.

Place flat fingers over the cheeks in front of the ears, and massage for at least a minute.

Place the palms of the hands on the forehead and the fingers on the scalp, and massage this area with large stationary circles for about one minute, about seven circles per minute.

Then, place the palms on the temples, between the forehead and ears, with the fingers on the scalp, and massage for about one minute, in seven circles.

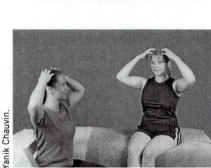

Massage the scalp on the top of the head for a minute. Be sure to move the scalp, not just the hair.

Next, place the palms of the hands behind the ears, with the fingers covering the back of the head, and massage the scalp for one minute, seven circles about seven seconds each.

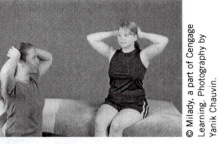

Place the fingers of both hands along the base of the skull and massage for about one minute, seven circles about seven seconds each.

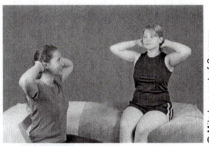

Finish by massaging the lymph nodes again, in reverse order:

Suboccipital nodes (base of the skull)

Pre- and post-auricular nodes

Submandibular and submental nodes

Cervical nodes

Supraclavicular nodes

STEP-BY-STEP   Self-Massage of the Upper Limbs

For this massage, it is probably most comfortable to lie down, propped up by a couple of pillows. Raise an arm overhead, supported by a pillow.

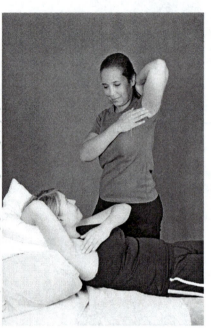

Place the fingers of the opposite hand deep into the center of the armpit and massage lightly for two or three minutes. Move the skin in stationary circles, about seven circles per minute, which is very slow.

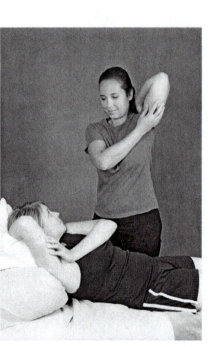

Next, place flat fingers just above the armpit on the arm and massage for two or three minutes, using stationary circles.

Reach under the pectoralis muscle in front of the armpit and massage for two or three minutes.

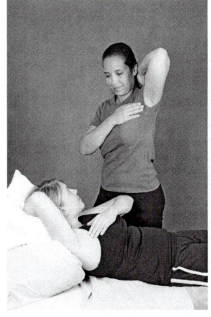

Reach under the latissimus dorsi muscle at the back of the armpit and massage the lymph nodes there for two or three minutes.

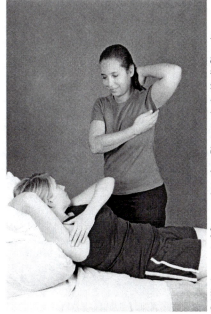

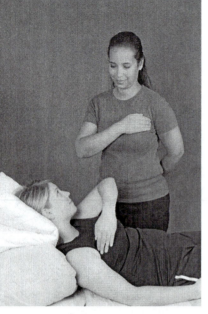

© Milady, a part of Cengage Learning. Photography by Yanik Chauvin.

Massage the chest wall around the outside of the breast. Place one hand above the breast and below the clavicle and massage for about one minute, using stationary circles, about seven circles per minute.

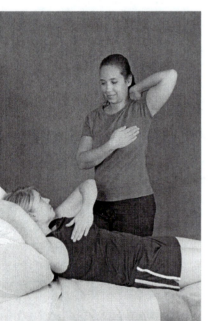

© Milady, a part of Cengage Learning. Photography by Yanik Chauvin.

Place the entire hand next to the outside of the breast and massage for one minute, using stationary circles.

Place the entire hand on the rib cage under the breast and massage for one minute.

Place the fingertips of both hands on the sternum and massage for one minute.

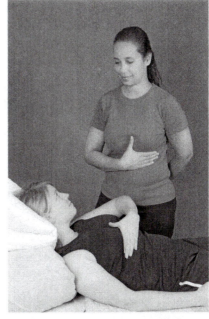

Massage the breast. Divide the breast into four sections and massage each section for about one minute, using stationary circles and repeating the circles seven times in a minute. Finish this section by brushing from the sternum over and around the breast toward the lymph nodes in the armpit.

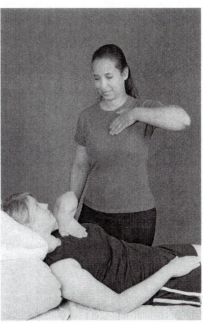

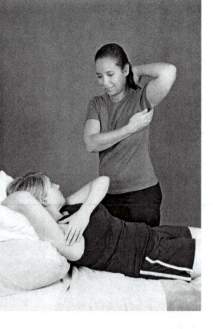

© Milady, a part of Cengage Learning. Photography by Yanik Chauvin.

Massage the upper arm. Lightly and very slowly, brush the lymph with fingertips toward the lymph nodes, from the elbow to the shoulder joint. Repeat each brush stroke seven or more times before moving to a new area on the upper arm.

Massage the lower arm. Lightly and very slowly, brush the lymph with fingertips toward the upper arm, from the wrist to the elbow. Repeat each brush stroke seven or more times before moving to a new area on the lower arm.

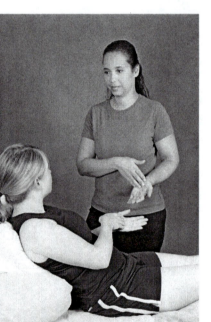

© Milady, a part of Cengage Learning. Photography by Yanik Chauvin.

Massage the hand. Use the fingertips of one hand to massage the pads in the palm of the other hand, using stationary circles, for about one minute. Wrap the fingers of the opposite hand around one of the fingers on the hand to be massaged, with the thumb on the section of the finger closest to the palm. Massage each finger for about one minute, using stationary circles, about seven circles per minute. Repeat for all fingers. Then massage the other hand and fingers.

With fingertips, repeat the brush strokes slowly from the hand to the shoulder. Finish by massaging the lymph nodes in the axilla again.

SELF-MASSAGING THE LOWER LIMBS

STEP-BY-STEP

Self-massage of the lower limbs can be a little awkward, especially if one lacks flexibility. However, it can still be very effective and should be attempted. To massage the inguinal nodes, lie down on a bed, face up, with the upper body supported by one or two pillows. Rest one hand gently over the top of the thigh, just below the inguinal ligament. Without pressing deeply into the tissue, try to locate the femoral pulse. Then, using the location of the pulse as another landmark, place one hand along the inguinal ligament, with the fingers reaching to the area where the femoral pulse was located. Using light pressure, move the skin around in a slow circle, taking about seven seconds to complete the circle. Repeat the circles for two to three minutes until there is a palpable change in the tissue. Moving in larger circles, the skin should feel softer, warmer, and more elastic.

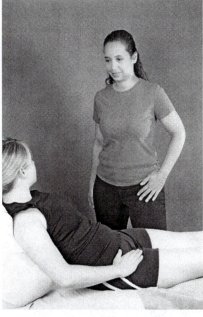

© Milady, a part of Cengage Learning. Photography by Yanik Chauvin.

Place two hands on the abdomen, between the inguinal ligament and the navel. Using both hands, move the skin of the abdomen in large circles, taking about seven seconds to complete a circle. Massage this area for two to three minutes. If the abdomen is large or the hands small, it might be necessary to massage the abdomen in sections. Cover the area from the midline of the trunk to the side seam, from the waist to the inguinal ligament, massaging each area at least one minute.

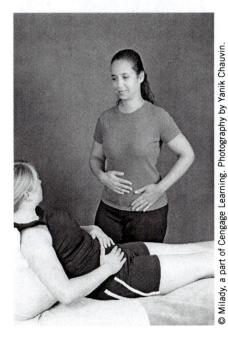

© Milady, a part of Cengage Learning. Photography by Yanik Chauvin.

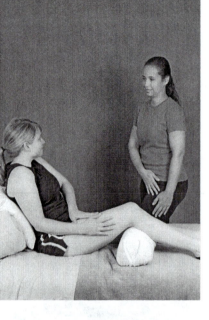

© Milady, a part of Cengage Learning. Photography by Yanik Chauvin.

To massage the leg, sit up enough to reach the entire thigh, placing pillows to support the back and elevate the knee with a small pillow. Place two hands on the upper thigh, near the inguinal ligament, covering the top and outside of the thigh. Move the skin in as large circles as possible, very slowly. Take about seven seconds to complete one circle, and repeat for at least one minute. Move down the thigh a hand's width and repeat. Work down the thigh to the knee.

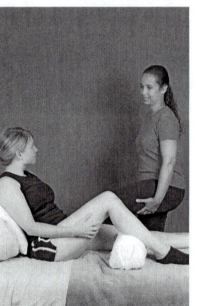

© Milady, a part of Cengage Learning. Photography by Yanik Chauvin.

Bend the knee more so that the back of the thigh is accessible. Placing the hands behind the thigh, move the skin in circles, taking about seven seconds to complete a circle. Repeat for at least one minute. Move the hands to another location on the back of the thigh, until the whole area has been massaged. Lightly grasp both sides of the knee and massage the area for at least one minute.

Remove the small pillow supporting the knee and extend the leg flat on the bed. Bending over to reach the lower leg, place both hands below the knee, wrapping around as much of the lower leg as possible. Move the skin in large, slow circles as before, taking at least one minute to massage. Move down the leg in small increments, working at least one minute on each area.

Covering the ankles with flat fingers, move the skin in slow circles for one minute. Massage the top of the foot with one hand, using slow circles, for about one minute. Massage the bottom of the foot in two steps: the ball of the foot, and then the heel pad. It is more difficult to move the skin on the sole of the foot, so it is tempting to use heavier pressure. Continue to use light pressure, about one ounce, and move the skin as well as possible in slow circles for about one minute.

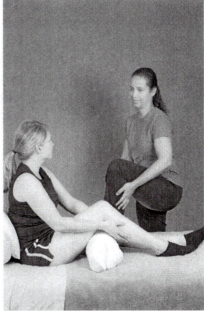

Massage by sliding the hands slowly from the foot to the knee, and repeat this movement seven times in one minute. Repeat on the back of the lower leg, sliding slowly from the heel to the knee seven times, very slowly with light pressure. Slide one or both hands from the knee to the hip, using light pressure, moving very slowly and repeating at least seven times.

Massage the inguinal lymph nodes again for two or three minutes.

TREATING SOFT-TISSUE INJURIES

For recent injuries that have begun to heal but are still swollen and painful, LDM is beneficial. First, make sure that the injury is examined to rule out underlying serious injuries, unless the injury is minor and has begun to heal, and pain is reduced. Do not massage over areas with open cuts, scratches, abrasions, or surgical incisions. Wait until these areas have healed to avoid infection.

Palpate the injured area and locate the outer edge of the painful area. Use your fingers to make small, slow circles, about seven seconds per circle, and repeat for at least one minute or until there is a palpable change in the tissue. Work in a circle around the edge of the injured area. Then move in a spiral pattern, going gradually toward the most painful area in the center. If the injury is very tender, this can take a long time. At the end of the session, pain should be reduced and bruising less visible.

If the injury is old, even years old, and completely healed but still swollen, a combination of connective tissue massage and LDM can help. There might be scars that are not visible; inflammation in the skin and muscles can result in scarring that can be felt, although it cannot be seen. To reduce scar tissue, first stretch the connective tissue. Use skin rolling, cross-fiber friction, or deep, slow strokes until the area is red and warm. Connective tissue massage should not be painful, but there will be a burning sensation when done correctly. Skin rolling is performed by picking up the skin between thumb and fingers and rolling the skin over the thumb with the fingers. Alternate hands so the movement is continuous along the tissue. Cross-fiber friction is performed by rubbing across or at right angles to scar tissue until a burning sensation is felt. To perform the deep, slow massage stroke that stretches the superficial fascia, press stiff fingers into the skin, then push slowly along the length of the scarred area with enough pressure to feel a burn in the tissues. Follow with LDM as described previously.

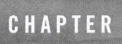

Healing Crisis

Although the concept of a healing crisis is not generally recognized outside alternative therapies, massage therapists and others in similar fields have experienced this phenomenon in their practices. Clients who begin health regimens that depart from their lifestyles may experience difficult periods. They may re-experience symptoms of previous illnesses, such as childhood asthma. They may report that they taste antibiotics, although they have taken none in years. They may start to ache in the area of an old injury. These experiences are temporary, but they can be alarming if the therapist does not prepare the client for the experience.

A healing crisis can happen to clients who are receiving one or a series of lymph drainage massage sessions. Therapists should tell clients that occasionally people experience a slight malaise, flu symptoms or other symptoms, after massage. Instruct the clients to drink fluids, rest, and in general, treat themselves as if they have the flu. A healing crisis is temporary and is accepted among alternative practitioners as a sign that the therapy is working. If the symptoms last longer than three days, the client may actually be ill and should seek treatment.

UNDERSTANDING THE HEALING CRISIS

The healing crisis is a purely non-medical empirical concept. The idea of the healing crisis is one of the underlying principles unique to alternative therapies that set those therapies apart from mainstream medical practice. In practical terms, the idea of a healing crisis refers to the experience clients sometimes have of feeling worse before they feel better, when they begin to adopt healthier lifestyles. Massage therapists and estheticians should be aware that their clients will sometimes experience healing crises following LDM. When they have been informed, clients generally feel positive about the experiences. Clients who have not been informed of the healing crisis can become alarmed, and feel that massage work somehow harmed them. Therefore, communication is crucial, but it is also important not to overemphasize the possibility of a healing crisis, because it does not happen to everyone.

The concept of a healing crisis derives from the belief that disease, particularly chronic disease, is caused by toxicity, and that toxicity is the result of both physical and emotional pollution that has accumulated in the human system over time. The symptoms the client experiences during the healing crisis can be both physical and emotional. At the physical level, toxicity is believed to be caused by years of inadequate diet that has polluted the system, as well as exposure to environmental pollutants over time such as pesticides, herbicides, heavy metals, PCBs, vinyl compounds, dioxin, bisphenol A, plastics, petroleum products, etc. It is also attributed to continual suppression of acute disease, through the overuse of pain medicine, antibiotics, and the like, which some alternative therapists believe will build toxicity in the system. Also, the overuse of any prescription medication can build toxicity in the body if these agents are stored in the liver over time.

The concept of the healing crisis was developed in an attempt to explain the symptoms that clients reported after massage, and was based on the understanding of physiological processes that existed at the time, as well as the observation by therapists that skilled touch readily activates both physical and nonphysical symptoms that can alarm the client. The truth is that lymph drainage massage affects the client on many levels. It does not simply remove fluid from tissues spaces and return it to the cardiovascular system. LDM affects the skin, muscles, the removal of waste, mood, pain, sleep and perhaps even the levels of medications in the bloodstream. As time goes on, medical research will clarify our understanding of how LDM affects all these processes in the body. In the meantime, it is important to reassure clients that these symptoms sometimes happen and are mostly benign.

Healing crises are to be taken in stride. Generally, clients enjoy LDM and afterward feel better, relaxed, and soothed. A healing crisis will not occur with every client or with every massage session. When a healing crisis does occur, it can begin spontaneously during the LDM session, or it can be precipitated by the work and occur later. The reaction may be physical (e.g., flu symptoms, shivering, mild nausea) or nonphysical (e.g., weeping, emotional release, visions). The healing crisis might involve releases on more than one level. For instance, the client may weep during the massage, remembering a childhood sorrow, then go home and suffer upper respiratory symptoms. When this kind of event occurs during a session, experienced practitioners realize that their responsibility is to remain with the client, quietly and sensitively, until the release is over.

With experience, practitioners will come to recognize clients who have greater potential for healing crises than others. Some clients are emotionally too unstable to weather the fallout of some treatments. Other clients may have simply neglected their health for so many years that a healing crisis is inevitable when they begin to change their lives, including receiving massage treatments. When in doubt, limit the length and frequency of lymph massage. Combine LDM with other massage techniques that are more generalized. Also, be prepared to refer clients to appropriate counselors or medical practitioners if they are having difficulty with memories or feelings experienced during or after the massage, or are feeling ill for more than three days after the session.

Chapter 1

1. Who was the first doctor to develop a method of lymph drainage massage?

    Alexander von Winiwater

2. Which doctor opened the first school offering training in lymph drainage massage?

    Dr. Johannes Asdonk

3. What is comprehensive decongestive therapy?

    Treatment for lymphedema disease that includes massage, bandaging, exercise and skin care.

4. What are the effects of LDM?

    LDM stimulates the movement of fluid out of tissue spaces, through the lymphatic system and back to the cardiovascular system. It stimulates lymph vessels to contract, moves tissue fluid away from areas of stagnation, stimulates the circulation of white blood cells throughout the body, and helps to reduce scar tissue. It is deeply relaxing, reduces pain, and improves sleep.

5. How is LDM performed?

    LDM mimics the lymphatic system and employs repetitive massage strokes at a precise speed, rhythm, and pressure.

6. What is the purpose of LDM?

    To enhance lymph circulation and immunity and maintain health on the one hand, and to treat chronic edema and lymphedema disease on the other hand.

7. What are the physiological effects of LDM?

    LDM stimulates lymph vessels to contract, pulls open the initial lymphatics, drains excess fluid and proteins from tissues, and returns fluid to the cardiovascular system.

8. What is edema?

    Edema is an abnormal accumulation of fluid in tissues such as the skin, connective tissue and muscles.

9. Compare and contrast LDM for the clinical setting and the wellness setting.

In a clinical setting, LDM is used after cosmetic surgery to reduce swelling, speed healing and reduce the development of scar tissue. It is used in the treatment of lymphedema disease, which is chronic obstructive edema that can develop after surgery, injury or radiation treatment. It is part of comprehensive decongestive therapy, along with non-elastic bandages, compression garments, exercise and skin care.

In the wellness setting, LDM is used to enhance the immune system by improving lymph circulation and increasing the distribution of leukocytes throughout the body. It is used to reduce edema, improve the appearance and health of the skin, reduce pain, stress and anxiety, and improve sleep.

10. What factors can cause edema?

    Obstruction, diet, inactivity, heart or kidney failure, hypothyroidism and other hormone imbalances, stress

11. What is primary lymphedema?

    Chronic edema due to congenital malformation of lymph and/or blood vessels.

12. What is secondary lymphedema?

    Secondary lymphedema is due to obstruction.

13. What factors or events can cause obstructive lymphedema?

    Surgery, injury, radiation therapy.

14. Describe some complications of lymphedema disease.

    Chronic edema, scar tissue, infection, lack of mobility, isolation and depression.

Chapter 2

1. Describe lymph. What is its source, and how does it differ from interstitial fluid?

    Lymph is the fluid in lymph vessels. It originates as plasma, extravasated from blood vessels into tissues. It is absorbed from the tissues into lymph vessels, and it has a higher protein concentration than interstitial fluid.

2. How do initial lymphatic vessels differ from lymph capillaries?

Initial lymphatics are made of a single layer of overlapping cells, attached by anchoring filaments to surrounding tissues. When tissue fluid pressure increases, the overlapping cells move apart, allowing tissue fluid to enter into the lymphatics. Lymph capillaries have smooth muscle cells in their walls and are able to contract, moving fluid through the capillaries toward larger vessels and toward lymph nodes.

3. What are lymphatic ducts? How many are there?

    The lymphatic ducts are the two largest lymph channels, the right lymphatic duct and the thoracic duct. They drain into the subclavian or internal jugular veins.

4. Describe a lymph node. How does it help protect against disease?

    Lymph nodes are small bean-shaped masses of lymph tissue located along the pathways of lymph vessels. They consist of fibrous coverings containing lymph cells and fibers, arranged into sections called sinuses. Afferent vessels attach to the nodes at various places; the efferent vessels emerge from a depression in the node called the hilus. Immune cells in the nodes analyze lymph fluid and recognize pathogens, stimulating a defensive reaction.

5. In what two ways do lymph capillaries differ from blood capillaries?

    Lymph capillaries have thinner walls and more valves than blood capillaries, and are connected to lymph nodes.

6. Into which large veins do the lymphatic ducts empty?

    The subclavian or internal jugular veins.

7. What is the function of the bicuspid valves in the lymph vessels?

    The bicuspid valves prevent backflow of lymph fluid.

8. The thoracic duct receives lymph fluid from which areas of the body?

The thoracic duct drains the lower extremities, abdomen and pelvis and the left upper trunk and arm, as well as the left side of the head and neck.

9. What is the difference between afferent and efferent lymph vessels?

    Afferent vessels empty fluid into lymph nodes; efferent vessels carry fluid out of nodes.

10. Where are the tonsils located, and how many are there?

    Tonsils are located in a ring around the opening to the digestive and respiratory tract. There are six tonsils.

11. What is the function of the tonsils?

    Tonsils are lymph nodes that destroy foreign cells when they enter the digestive and respiratory tracts.

12. How do tonsils differ from other lymph nodes?

    Tonsils don't have afferent vessels. Instead, they analyze material passing through the area they protect, defending against pathogens that are inhaled or ingested.

13. Which lymphatic organ stores blood? What are its other functions?

    The spleen filters and stores blood. It destroys old red blood cells and protects against pathogens circulating in blood.

14. Where is the thymus located?

    The thymus is located under the superior end of the sternum.

15. What role does the thymus play in the lymphatic system?

    The thymus is an endocrine gland consisting of connective tissue and lymph tissue. It produces a hormone that helps T-cells mature, and it helps with newborn infants' immunity.

16. Describe the location of lymph nodules and the purpose they serve.

    Lymph nodules are small collections of lymph tissue

located in the mucus membrane that lines the respiratory and digestive tracts.

Chapter 3

1. List at least three factors that affect lymph circulation.

    Respiration, exercise, lymphatic pump capability, gravity and massage.

2. What are the two stages of lymph circulation?

    Absorption into initial lymphatics, and propulsion through lymph vessels.

3. Describe differences between the structure of lymph and blood vessels.

    Blood vessels have a well-defined basement membrane, which is an outer wall of connective tissue that gives them structure and resilience. These blood vessel membranes are fenestrated, or honeycombed with windows, through which plasma, proteins, and red blood cells escape from the blood to the cell spaces in tissues and organs. Lymph vessels, in contrast, are more loosely structured. Because of this, proteins and other components of tissue fluid can enter the lymphatic system easily. They enter through gaps between endothelial cells in the initial lymphatics.

4. What is the lymphatic pump?

    It is the action of smooth muscle cells in the walls of the lymphangions contracting, creating a wave-like propulsion of lymph from tissue spaces into the lymphatics and toward the lymph nodes.

5. Describe the effects of exercise on lymph circulation.

    During exercise, lymphatic circulation inside muscles increases up to 15 times the resting rate. At first, the lymphatic fluid from the muscles is full of proteins, dead red blood cells, and waste material from the muscle cells. As exercise continues, the muscles continue to alternately contract and relax, propelling lymph through the vessels and pulling fluid from the muscle tissues that becomes progressively less infiltrated with waste. Exercise has the effect of scrubbing the muscles clean.

6. The lymphatic system is part of what larger system?

The cardiovascular system.

Chapter 4

1. What are the main functions of the lymphatic system?

Immunity, fluid balance, removal of proteins from tissues, distribution of dietary fat, and cleanup of damaged tissues after an injury.

2. Why is it important for protein to be removed from tissues, and why are the blood vessels unable to absorb proteins from tissues?

Left in the tissues, proteins can trigger an inflammatory response and the side effects of pain, swelling, and scar tissue. As a result of inflammation, scar tissue builds up in the area, making the tissues more coarse and less flexible.

3. How does dietary fat enter the bloodstream and pass through the heart?

Lymph vessels called lacteals are located in the lining of the small intestine. Emulsified dietary fat enters the lacteals and is transported to the intestinal lymphatic trunk, and then to the cisterna chyli at the base of the thoracic duct. Lymph and dietary fat travel through the thoracic duct and empty into the venous system near the heart.

4. What role does the lymphatic system play when there is an injury to a tissue like the skin or muscles?

Blood circulation in the area increases, and capillaries become more permeable. More fluid is released into the damaged area, bringing with it immune cells

and fibers that start to wall off the area and destroy any dangerous microorganisms. The pressure difference between the fluid-filled tissues and the lymphatic vessels creates a slight vacuum that pulls debris from the injury, including dead cells, microorganisms, and foreign particles, into the initial lymphatics and eventually to the lymph nodes, where it is destroyed.

5. What role does the lymphatic system play when someone is exposed to a disease-causing microorganism?

Lymph nodes filter lymph and the spleen filters blood. These organs contain lymphocytes that can recognize and destroy microorganisms which threaten the organism.

6. How does the lymphatic system affect blood volume?

Tissue fluid is absorbed into the lymphatic system and returned to the cardiovascular system.

7. What is the most important function of the lymphatic system?

Immunity.

Chapter 5

1. How does nonspecific immunity differ from specific immunity?

Nonspecific immunity is built into the human body at birth. It consists of anatomical barriers such as the skin, mechanical methods of resistance such as the cilia that line the respiratory tract, receptors that recognize molecular patterns shared by a variety of antigens, non-specific chemicals on the skin and in tears, mucus and saliva that function to keep out pathogens, as well as phagocytosis, inflammation and fever. Unlike acquired immunity, the innate immune responses do not "learn" from repeated exposure

to a given infection, so they don't improve over time.

2. Specific immunity depends on what two factors?

The body's ability to recognize harmful foreign cells and create antibodies.

3. What is an antibody?

Antibodies are proteins produced by immune cells in response to antigens. Antibodies bind to antigens, neutralizing them.

4. What is an antigen?

A disease-causing organism such as a bacteria or virus, or a substance that causes an allergic reaction.

5. How does inflammation protect the body from disease?

By stimulating the body's defenses: blood circulation increases, carrying immune cells toward the injury or infection. Immune cells battle against foreign invaders, and fibers begin the process of rebuilding damaged tissue and walling off infection.

6. In what four ways can specific immunity be acquired?

By exposure to pathogens, either naturally or through vaccination; also by transfer of antibodies either naturally or through the injection of another person's antibodies.

7. Give two examples of nonspecific immunity.

Nonspecific immunity occurs in a generic way when the skin acts as a barrier to disease, when chemicals on the skin, in mucus, and in tears fight against pathogenic invaders, and when inflammation occurs in response to bacteria or viruses.

8. Describe three lymphocytes.

Natural killer cells, B- and T-lymphocytes.

9. Is there a difference between a monocyte and a macrophage?

Monocytes are immature macrophages that travel in blood and lymph. As they mature, they increase dramatically in size.

10. Give an example of mechanical resistance to disease.

The skin barrier, and the cilia that line the respiratory tract provide mechanical resistance to disease.

11. Give an example of chemical resistance.

Lysozyme in tears and saliva, sebum on skin, and mucus on membranes are chemicals that prevent invaders from entering the body. Internally, interferon acts to prevent viral replication in the body's cells.

Chapter 6

1. How does dietary salt intake contribute to edema?

Increased dietary salt causes the body to retain water so that a constant and specific ratio of salt to water can be maintained.

2. What are the common causes of obstructive edema?

Scar tissue from injury, surgery, radiation, or infection.

3. How does exercise affect lymph circulation in muscles?

Exercise increases the circulation of lymph inside muscles up to 15 times the resting rate.

4. Besides obstruction, what other factors may contribute to edema?

Diet, allergies, medications, inactivity, position (sitting or standing too long without movement).

5. Describe pitting edema.

Pitting edema is characterized by a depression that remains after pressing into the tissue with a fingertip, and then removing the pressure.

6. What tissue changes occur with chronic edema?

Fibrosis develops, and the tissue becomes harder, colder, thicker and coarser due to the buildup of fibers in the area.

7. What is the long-term outlook for lymphedema disease?

Lymphedema disease is a lifelong condition.

8. What are the possible complications of chronic lymphedema disease?

Infection could occur, causing more scar tissue; there is also the possibility that a limb would have to be amputated.

9. How is lymphedema disease treated?

LDM, bandaging, exercise and scrupulous skin care.

10. What factors can cause edema?

Diet, allergies, injury, surgery, radiation, infection, inactivity, position.

11. What is primary lymphedema disease?

Primary lymphedema disease is a congenital condition possibly caused by a malformation of blood or lymph vessels.

12. What is secondary lymphedema disease?

Secondary lymphedema disease is chronic obstruction of lymph vessels, which inhibits their ability to absorb interstitial fluid into the lymphatic system, resulting in chronic edema.

13. What factors or events can cause obstructive lymphedema?

Injury, surgery, radiation, or infection.

14. Describe some complications of lymphedema.

Infection is a serious complication, since the edematous area heals more slowly because lymph circulation is inhibited. Lymphedema disease causes

pain, reduces mobility, limits daily activities and contributes to depression.

Chapter 8

1. What is the purpose of moving the skin when applying LDM?

To open the flaps of the initial lymphatics and allow fluid to enter the lymphatic vessels.

2. What is the optimal pressure for LDM?

Half an ounce to eight ounces of pressure per square inch.

3. Why is it important to repeat massage strokes when performing LDM, and what is the recommended rate?

There are six to ten contractions of the peripheral lymphatics per minute. Repeating the massage strokes at this rate for at least a minute at each location triggers rhythmic contractions in the vessels, establishing normal circulation.

4. In what direction is the therapist trying to move the lymph when performing LDM?

c. Toward the lymph nodes.

5. What is the basic pattern or order of movements in LDM?

Massage over the lymph nodes first. Then massage proximal to distal, massaging near the lymph nodes and then gradually moving toward the margins of the lymphotomes and the distal ends of the limbs.

6. What can happen if the lymph nodes are not massaged before massaging an edematous area?

Fluid can accumulate in the tissues surrounding the lymph nodes, causing discomfort.

7. Why is slow, rhythmic repetition of strokes so important?

d. All of the above

8. What are watersheds?

The margins of the lympho-tomes, which are the regions drained by the inguinal and axillary lymph nodes.

9. From memory, draw a sketch of the pattern of lymph drainage to the trunk and extremities. Include the watersheds and the location of lymph nodes.

10. Because of the watersheds, lymph can be directed around obstructions and drained toward the nodes of the unaffected side of the body.

   a. True

11. Why is the well or unaffected side massaged first when working with obstructive edema?

   To stimulate normal lymph drainage, which will then provide a place that the fluid can go when massaging the obstructed side.

12. What is the basic movement or stroke in LDM?

   A stationary circle.

13. Why is the ability to focus and concentrate important in LDM? How can one increase the ability to concentrate?

   The ability to focus and concentrate helps the therapist recognize subtle clues in the tissue that signify that the fluid is moving away from the area, and it allows the therapist to follow the movement of lymph across the body.

   To increase concentration, practice focusing, try not to chat with your client while you are working, eliminate distractions, count the number of repetitions, and keep track of the seconds that elapse for each repetition.

14. What is the proper stance for the therapist when performing LDM standing up? When seated?

   Stand with your weight on both feet, knees slightly bent, and keep the back straight. Stay near the area you are working on, rather than leaning over and stretching awkwardly to reach the area. When seated, position your spine over your hips, sit as close to the massage table as you can, and keep both feet on the floor.

Chapter 14

1. Explain the importance of the setting for the massage.

   The setting for the massage, the room itself, music, other sounds, comfortable table and decor, help the client relax and induce trust.

2. What elements of the massage produce a meditative state?

   Lymph drainage massage is slow, repetitive and gentle.

3. Why is it important to set boundaries in a massage? What boundaries could you set that help to protect your client?

   Setting professional boundaries protects the client and therapist from the possible confusion of a dual relationship, shows the therapist's respect for the client's rights and needs and keeps the relationship professional.

4. What can occur when a client enters a relaxed dream state during the massage?

   The client can remember past events, uncomfortable feelings may arise, the client may become disoriented as to time and place.

5. What mistakes might you make with a client if you don't honor your own boundaries and your client's boundaries when the client is in a relaxed dream state?

   You might be tempted to interpret the experience for the client, counsel the client about the experience or react inappropriately to the client's experience because of your own experiences.

6. What subtle responses can happen during a lymph drainage massage that might surprise the client or the therapist?

   Clients who are experiencing emotional release can feel sad, angry, afraid, silly, libidinous, or child-like. The massage session may be further complicated if the client attempts to repress or hold in the emotional memories because he or she feels the emotions are unacceptable, for instance if the client is experiencing fear or anger. The client may feel tremendously sad and not know why. The client may become sexually aroused and either act out inappropriately or feel shame and embarrassment. The client may be afraid of ridicule or ostracism.

7. How should a therapist or esthetician handle a client's emotional release?

   The therapist's job is to communicate, listen, and not become involved. First assure the client that these feelings are normal; everyone has feelings trapped in muscles and when the muscles are released, the feelings arise. Assure the client that the feeling will go away, and that it is a historical feeling. It is related to events in the past, not the present.

8. How would you handle it if your client begins to seem angry during a massage?

   Ask the client what is happening and how does he/she feel.

9. How would you handle it if your client begins to cry during a massage?

   Reassure the client that it is all right to cry, hand the client some tissue, refrain from asking questions or interpreting the experience.

Preface

1. Gasparo Asselli described the lymph vessels in a dog in 1622; Johann Vesling observed human lymph vessels in 1624. William Harvey described human blood circulation in 1628.
2. Chikly B., MD. *Silent Waves: The Theory and Practice of Lymph Drainage Therapy.* Scottsdale, AZ: IHH Publishing; 2001:12.
3. National Lymphedema Network, 21 Post St., Suite 404, San Francisco, CA 94115, http://www.lymphnet.org. Accessed June 2011.
4. DeGodoy JMP. Preliminary evaluation of a new, more simplified physiotherapy technique for lymphatic drainage. *Lymphology.* 2002;35:91–93.

Chapter One

1. Kirby RM, Basit A, Nguyen QT, Jaipersad A, Billingham R. Three stage axillary lymphatic massage optimizes sentinel lymph node localisation using blue dye. *Int Semin Surg Oncol.* 2007;4:30.
2. Casley-Smith JR, Boris M, Weindorf S, Lasinski B. Treatment for lymphedema of the arm—The Casley-Smith method: a noninvasive method produces continued reduction. *Cancer.* 1998;83(12 Suppl American):2843-60.
3. Winiwater F. Das Elephantiasis. "*Deutsche Chirugie.*" Stuttgart: Enke; 1892:23.
4. Wittlinger H, Wittlinger G. *Textbook of Dr. Vodder's Manual Lymph Drainage, Vol 1: Basic Course,* 3rd ed. Heidelberg: Haug; 1982.
5. Foldi E. Comprehensive lymphedema treatment center. *Lymphology.* 1994;27:505–7.
6. Foldi M. Treatment of lymphedema. *Lymphology.* 1994;27(1):1–5.
7. Casley-Smith JR, Casley-Smith JR. Modern treatment of lymphoedema II: the benzopyrones. *Australas J Dermatol.* 1992;33(2):6974.
8. Zuther JE. *Lymphedema Management: The Comprehensive Guide for Practitioners.* New York: Thieme Medical Publishers; 2005.

9. Olszewski WL (ed.). *Lymph Stasis: Pathophysiology, Diagnosis, and Treatment.* Boca Raton, FL: CRC Press; 1991.
10. Casley-Smith, J.R. Lymphatic manifesto. Lymphology. 1984;17, 109-110

Chapter Three

1. O'Morchoe CCC, O'Morchoe PJ. Differences in lymphatic and blood capillary permeability: ultrastructural-functional correlations. *Lymphology.* 1987;20:205–209.
2. Solito R, Alessandrini C, Fruschelli M, Pucci AM, Gerli R. An immunological correlation between the anchoring filaments of initial lymph vessels and the neighboring elastic fibers: a unified morphofunctional concept. *Lymphology.* 1997;30(4):194–202.
3. Ryan TJ. The skin and its response to movement. *Lymphology.* 1998;31(3):128–129.
4. Castenholz A. Functional microanatomy of initial lymphatics with special consideration of the extracellular matrix. *Lymphology.* 1998;31:101–118.
5. Witte CL, Witte MH. Contrasting patterns of lymphatic and blood circulatory disorders. *Lymphology.* 1987;20:171–78.
6. Reddy NP. Lymph circulation: physiology, pharmacology, and biomechanics. *CRC Critical Reviews in Biomedical Engineering.* 1986;14(1):45–91.
7. Szuba A, Rockson SG. Lymphedema: anatomy, physiology and pathogenesis. *Vasc Med.* 1997;2(4):321–6.
8. Casley-Smith JR. Lymphatic manifesto. *Lymphology.* 1984;17:109–10.
9. Hall JG, Morris B, Woolley G. Intrinsic rhythmic propulsion of lymph in the unanaesthetized sheep. *J Physiol.* 1965;180(2):336–49.
10. Guyton AC. *Textbook of Medical Physiology,* 6th ed. Philadelphia: Saunders; 1981.
11. *Lymphedema Therapy*: Lymphedema and Exercises. http://**www.lymphedema-therapy.com/**

lymphedema-exercise.html
Accessed June 2011.

12. National Lymphedema Network, 21 Post St., Suite 404, San Francisco, CA 94115, http://www.lymphnet.org. *Position Statement of The National Lymphedema Network, Topic: Exercise,* http://www.lymphnet.org/pdfDocs/nlnexercise.pdf Accessed June 2011.

13. Desai PV, Williams A Jr, Prajapati PR, Downey HF. Lymph flow in instrumented dogs varies with exercise intensity. *Lymphat Res Biol.* 2010;8 (3):143–8.

14. Ryan TJ. The skin and its response to movement. *Lymphology.* 1998;31(3):128–129.

15. Parsons RJ, McMaster PD. The effect of the pulse upon the formation and flow of lymph. *J Exp Med.* 1938;68(3):353–76.

16. Caenar JS, Pflug JJ, Reig NO, Taylor LM. Lymphatic pressures and the flow of lymph. *Br J Plast Surg.* 1970;23:205.

17. McMaster PD. Changes in the cutaneous lymphatics of human beings and in the lymph flow under normal and pathological conditions. *J Exp Med.* 1937;65(3):347–72.

Chapter Four

1. Casley-Smith JR. Lymphatic manifesto. *Lymphology.* 1984;17:109–110.

2. Yoffey JM, Courtice FC. *Lymphatics, Lymph, and Lymphomyeloid Complex.* New York: Academic Press; 1970.

3. Olszewski WL. Continuing discovery of the lymphatic system in the 21st century: a brief overview of the past. *Lymphology.* 2002;35(3):102–103.

4. Ibid.

Chapter Six

1. Casley-Smith JR. Lymphatic manifesto. *Lymphology.* 1984;17:109–110.

2. Olszewski WL, Ambujam PJ, Zaleska M, Cakala M. Where do lymph and tissue fluid accumulate in lymphedema of the lower limbs caused by obliteration of lymphatic collectors? *Lymphology.* 2009;42(3):105–11.

3. Olszewski WL, Jain P, Ambujam G, Zaleska M, Cakala M. Topography of accumulation of stagnant lymph and tissue fluid in soft tissues of human lymphedematous lower limbs. *Lymphat Res Biol.* 2009;7(4):239–45.

4. Linda Barufaldi, D.C., private communication.

5. Casley-Smith (1984).

6. Witte CL, Witte MH. Contrasting patterns of lymphatic and blood circulatory disorders. *Lymphology.* 1987;20:171–178.

7. Brorson H, Ohlin K, Olsson G, Nilsson M. Adipose tissue dominates chronic arm lymphedema following breast cancer: an analysis using volume rendered CT images. *Lymphat Res Biol.* 2006;4(4):199–210.

8. Desai PV, Williams A Jr, Prajapati PR, Downey, HF. Lymph flow in instrumented dogs varies with exercise intensity. *Lymphat Res Biol.* 2010;8(3):143–8.

9. Position Statement Of The National Lymphedema Network. Topic: Exercise **http://www.lymphnet.org/pdfDocs/nlnexercise.pdf.** Accessed June 2011.

10. Browse NL, Stewart G. Lymphoedema: pathophysiology and classification. *J Cardiovasc Surg* (Torino). 1985;26(2):91–106.

11. Weissleder H, Schuchhardt C (eds.). *Lymphedema Diagnosis and Therapy.* Bonn: Kagerer Kommunikation; 1997.

12. The diagnosis and treatment of peripheral lymphedema. 2009 consensus document of the International Society of Lymphology. *Lymphology.* 2009;42:53–54.

13. Kerchner K, Fleischer A., Yosipovitch G. Lower extremity lymphedema update: pathophysiology, diagnosis, and treatment guidelines. J Am Acad Dermatol. 2008;59: 324–331

Chapter Seven

1. Foldi E. Massage and damage to lymphatics. *Lymphology.* 1995;28(1):1–3.

2. Werner R, Benjamin B. *A Massage Therapist's Guide to Pathology.* Baltimore: Williams & Wilkins; 1998.

3. Burch S. *Recognizing Health and Illness.* Lawrence, KS: Health Positive! Publishing; 1997.

4. Wittlinger H, Wittlinger G. *Introduction to Dr. Vodder's Manual Lymph Drainage.* Heidelberg: Haug Verlag; 1982.

Chapter Eight

1. Caenar et al. (1970).
2. Parsons & McMaster (1938).
3. McMaster (1946).
4. Olszewski & Engeset (1979).
5. Wang & Zhong (1985).
6. J. M. P. de Godoy, F. Batigalia, M. de F. G. Godoy. Preliminary evaluation of a new, more simplified physiotherapy technique for lymphatic drainage. Lymphology, 35(2), 91–93.
7. Ryan, T. J. (1998). Lymphology, 128–129.
8. Wittlinger, H., & Wittlinger, G. (1982).
9. Wittlinger, H., & Wittlinger, G. (1998).
10. Mislin (1976).
11. Foldi, E: Editorial: Massage and Damage to Lymphatics. Lymphology 28 (1995) 1–3.
12. Eliska, O. and Eliskova, M.: Are Peripheral Lymphatics Damaged by High Pressure Manual Massage? Lymphology 28 (1995) 21–30.
13. Olszewski & Engeset (1979 and 1980).

14. RM Kirby, A Basit, QT Nguyen, A Jaipersad, R Billingham; Three Stage Axillary Lymphatic Massage Optimizes Sentinel Lymph Node Localisation Using Blue Dye; Int Semin Surg Oncl; 2007, 4:30.
15. Olszewski & Engeset (1979).
16. Olszewski, W. L. (ed.). (1991). Lymph stasis. 473.

Chapter Thirteen

1. Hodge LM, Bearden MK, Schander A, Huff JB, Williams AG Jr, King HH, Downey HF. Lymphatic pump treatment mobilizes leukocytes from the gut associated lymphoid tissue into lymph. *Lymphat Res Biol.* 2010;8(2):103–10.
2. Hodge LM, King HH, Williams AG Jr, Reder SJ, Belavadi T, Simecka JW, Stoll ST, Downey HF. Abdominal lymphatic pump treatment increases leukocyte count and flux in thoracic duct lymph. *Lymphat Res Biol.* 2007;5(2):127–33.

Chapter Fourteen

1. Leichtman R. Personal communication to Judy Dean; 2001.

Chapter Fifteen

1. Wang X, Ostberg JR, Repasky EA. Effect of fever-like whole-body hyperthermia on lymphocyte spectrin distribution, protein kinase C activity, and uropod formation. *J Immunol.* 1999;162(6):3378–87.
2. Duff GW. Is fever beneficial to the host: a clinical perspective. *Yale J Biol Med.* 1986;59(2):125–30.
3. Sypek JP, Burreson EM. Influence of temperature on the immune response of juvenile summer flounder, *Paralichthys dentatus*, and its role in the elimination of *Trypanoplasma bullocki* infections. *Dev Com Immunol.* 1983;7(2):277–86.
4. Kluger MJ, Ringler DH, Anver MR. Fever and survival. *Science.* 1975;188(4184):166–8.
5. Covert JB, Reynolds WW. Survival value of fever in fish. *Nature.* 1977; 267(5606):43–5.
6. Kappel M, Stadeager C, Tvede N, Galbo H, Pedersen BK. Effects of in vivo hyperthermia on natural killer cell activity, in vitro proliferative responses and blood mononuclear cell subpopulations. *Clin Exp Immunol.* 1991;84(1):175–80.
7. Duff GW, Durum SK. Fever and immunoregulation: hyperthermia, interleukins 1 and 2, and T-cell proliferation. *Yale J Biol Med.* 1982;55(5-6):437–42.
8. Duff GW, Durum SK. T cell proliferation induced by interleukin 1 is greatly increased by hyperthermia. *Clin Res.* 1982;30:694.
9. Wang WC, Goldman LM, Schleider DM, Appenheimer MM, Subjeck JR, Repasky EA, Evans SS. Fever-range hyperthermia enhances L-selectin-dependent adhesion of lymphocytes to vascular endothelium. *J Immunol.* 1998;160(2):961–9.
10. Lefor AT, Foster CE 3rd, Sartor W, Engbrecht B, Fabian DF, Silverman D. Hyperthermia increases intercellular adhesion molecule-1 expression and lymphocyte adhesion to endothelial cells. *Surgery.* 1994;116(2):214–20.
11. Burd R, Dziedzec TS, Xu Y, Caligiuri MA, Subjeck JR, Repasky EA. Tumor cell apoptosis, lymphocyte recruitment and tumor vascular changes are induced by low temperature, long duration whole body hyperthermia. *J Cell Physiol.* 1998;177(1):137–47.
12. Touch Therapy Institute. http://www.miami.edu/touch-research/index.html. Accessed June 2011.

Abdomen The part of the trunk between the ribs and the pelvis.

Abdominal aorta The part of the largest artery in the body that is located in the abdomen.

Abdominopelvic cavity Portion of the ventral cavity inferior to the diaphragm muscle, containing the liver and gallbladder, kidneys, spleen, stomach, intestines and pelvic organs.

Absorption Movement of dietary nutrients from the digestive tract into the lymphatic and cardiovascular systems.

Acquired Immune Deficiency Syndrome (AIDS) A group of diseases caused by the human immunodeficiency virus.

Acquired/Active immunity The ability to resist disease, which comes from the presence of antibodies developed after exposure to disease pathogens or their antigens. Natural acquired immunity depends on direct exposure to disease; artificial acquired immunity results from vaccination with weakened pathogens. Passive acquired immunity is the transfer of antibodies from a mother to a baby in the womb, or after birth, through breast milk. Artificial passive immunity is the transfer of active antibodies from a healthy person to a person who is not able to develop antibodies.

Adenoid Pharyngeal tonsil; the mass of lymphoid tissue at the back of the throat.

Adipose tissue Loose connective tissue containing fat cells.

Afferent vessel Lymphatic vessel that carries lymph to a lymph node; *see also efferent vessels.*

Aggregated lymph nodules Clusters of lymph tissue in the intestine and appendix that respond to the presence of antigens; also called Peyer's patches.

Anchoring filament An elastic fiber that connects the endothelial cell membrane of lymph vessels to the surrounding tissues.

Antibody A protein molecule produced by B-cells in response to antigens (disease- or allergy-causing agents); it destroys antigens.

Antigen A disease-causing substance such as a virus, bacteria, fungus or parasite; also pollen, food.

Aorta Largest artery in the body.

Aponeurosis A tendon, in the form of a wide, flat sheet of connective tissue that attaches to a flat muscle.

Areolar tissue Loose, irregularly arranged tissue that is the most common connective tissue in the body. It attaches the skin to the underlying tissue, cushions and protects organs, and holds them in place.

Autoimmune disease A condition in which the immune system attacks the body's own tissues. The immune system fails to recognize self-cells and attacks them as if they were invaders.

Axilla Armpit

Axillary nodes— Lymph nodes found in the armpit that drain the lymph channels from the breast.

B-cell A lymphocyte that produces antibodies; also called B-lymphocyte.

Basement membrane Connective tissue that attaches epithelial cells to surrounding tissues and to each other. Surrounds organs and vessels, providing support.

Basophil A type of white blood cell involved in allergic reactions and inflammation; a phagocytic leukocyte.

Bronchomediastinal lymphatic trunk The lymphatic vessel which drains lymph from the lungs, heart, diaphragm, the upper portion of the liver, and the rest of the thoracic cavity.

Capillary Microscopic, permeable blood vessel that delivers nutrients and oxygen to tissue cells, and absorbs metabolic waste and carbon dioxide from tissue fluid.

Cell-mediated immunity An immune response involving T-cells that attack pathogens and trigger the humoral immune response.

Cellulite Rippled and dimpled appearance of the skin, usually found on the abdomen, upper legs and buttocks as well as the back of the upper arms, due to the abnormal structure of the connective tissue surrounding the fat cells.

Cervical nodes Lymph nodes located in the neck that receive fluid from the head and neck and convey it to the jugular lymphatic trunk.

Chemical resistance Resistance due to nonspecific antiviral and antibacterial substances produced by the body.

Chyle A milky fluid consisting of digested dietary fat droplets and lymph.

Cisterna chyli A dilated sac at the lower end of the thoracic duct that receives and temporarily stores lymph as it travels upward from the lower body. Lymph from the lumbar lymphatic trunks and the intestinal lymphatic trunk flow into it, and it forms the primary lymph vessel that transports lymph and chyle from the abdomen to the subclavian and jugular veins. It is a reservoir that occurs inconsistently—not all people have it.

Connective tissue The most common type of tissue in the human body, consisting of cells, fibers and a gel-like matrix. It supports, anchors, connects, and gives structure to various parts of the body.

Contracture— A permanent tightening and hardening of muscles, tendons or other tissues that prevents normal movement of the associated body part, and can cause permanent deformity. A contracture develops when the normally elastic connective tissues are replaced by inelastic fibrous tissue. This makes the affected area resistant to stretching and prevents normal movement.

Debulking— General term used for surgeries in which subcutaneous tissue is removed from a lymphedemous limb.

Edema Condition in which excess interstitial fluid saturates the tissues, causing swelling.

Efferent vessels A lymph vessel that carries lymph *from* a lymph node. (Compare to an afferent vessel, which is a vessel that carries lymph *to* a lymph node). It is a one-way vessel leading out of a lymph node that carries lymph fluid toward the largest lymph vessels, the lymph trunks and ducts.

Elephantiasis Scarring of lymphatic vessels and/or nodes that causes obstruction of lymph flow, resulting in an enlarged limb (usually the leg and genital region); caused by filariasis.

Endothelial cells Simple squamous cells that line blood and lymph vessels.

Epithelial cells Cells found in the skin and on the surfaces of organs, as well as lining hollow structures such as the intestines, blood, and lymph vessels. Epithelial cells give structure and support, and are permeable so that fluids can pass into and out of organs, vessels, and tissues.

Erythrocyte A mature red blood cell.

Fibrosis The formation of fibrous tissue in response to damage or as a repair process; it may occur as a result of medical treatment and/or disease. In lymphedema disease, it causes a hardening of the limb which restricts the circulation of lymph and can lead to infections and weeping sores.

Fibrotic Pertaining to or characterized by fibrosis.

Flap valves Loosely overlapping lymphatic endothelial cells that form the walls of unidirectional valves inside the lymphatic capillaries. They are attached to surrounding structures with fibers that stretch and relax the capillaries, which causes the flap valves to separate and allow fluid to enter the lymph capillaries.

Humoral immunity An immune response that depends on the secretion and circulation of antibodies.

Immune system Lymph cells, tissues, and organs that provide a defense against foreign organisms and substances.

Immunity The body's ability to defend itself against damage from invading organisms such as viruses, bacteria, fungi and parasites.

Inflammation A defensive reaction involving cells and chemicals in response to injury or a physical, chemical, or biological agent that damages cells.

Interstitial fluid The fluid between cells in tissues, which is very similar in composition to lymph. It is the main component of the extracellular fluid.

Interstitial space The areas surrounding the cells of a given tissue that are filled with interstitial fluid; also known as tissue space.

Intestinal lymphatic trunk A lymph vessel that receives lymph fluid from the intestines, abdomen, pancreas and spleen, and that conveys fluid toward the cisterna chyli and thoracic duct.

Jugular lymphatic trunk Bilateral lymph vessel that receives lymph fluid from the cervical nodes and supraclavicular nodes, and conveys the fluid to the thoracic or right lymphatic duct.

Lacteal A specialized lymphatic vessel in the intestine that transports chyle (digested fat) to the cisterna chyli.

Leukocyte A scavenger white blood cell that attacks foreign cells and foreign matter in the tissues and bloodstream.

Lumbar lymphatic trunk A lymph vessel that receives lymph from one of the lower extremities and pelvis, and conveys it to the cisterna chyli and thoracic duct. There are two lumbar lymphatic trunks.

Lymph A clear or yellowish fluid that is absorbed from body tissues into the lymphatic system, where it passes through lymph nodes and into lymph vessels before being returned to the blood circulation. The fluid contains white blood cells, a few red blood cells, proteins, microorganisms, and microscopic particles.

Lymph drainage massage (LDM) A gentle, rhythmic style of massage that mimics the action of the lymphatic system using precise rhythm and pressure to reduce edema.

Lymph nodes Small (1–25 mm in diameter), bean-shaped masses of lymph tissue located along the pathway of lymphatic vessels that are the main source of lymphocytes. They consist of fibrous coverings containing lymph cells and fibers arranged into sinuses. There are usually small depressions on one side called hila, where efferent vessels emerge from the node; afferent vessels attach to the lymph node at various points around the periphery of the node.

Lymph nodule A spherical mass of lymphoid cells in the mucus membrane that lines the tonsils, spleen and thymus.

Lymph stasis Blockage of lymph flow, leading to an abnormal accumulation of fluid in tissues.

Lymphadenopathy Any disease that affects the lymph nodes.

Lymphangiography A type of medical imaging which uses dye to make the lymphatic vessels and nodes visible on an X-ray.

Lymphangion A muscular segment of the lymph vessels with bicuspid valves at each end to propel lymph forward and prevent lymph backflow; the functional unit of a lymph vessel.

Lymphatic capillaries The smallest vessels in the lymphatic system. These tiny capillaries occur throughout the body and absorb fluid from the tissues. They are very porous, with little or no basement membrane, consist of one layer of endothelial cells, and are closed at one end. They drain excess tissue fluids from around the cells, filter it, and then return it to venous circulation.

Lymphatic duct One of the two largest lymph vessels—the right lymphatic duct and the thoracic duct.

Lymphatic pump Spontaneous contraction of the smooth muscle cells in the walls of lymph vessels, which has the effect of propelling lymph.

Lymphatic system Consists of lymph, lymph tissue, lymph vessels, nodes, ducts, spleen, thymus, bone marrow and tonsils. The purpose of this system is to move fluid out of the tissue spaces and into the lymph vessels, where it is filtered by lymph nodes before returning to the blood circulatory system.

Lymphatic tissue A network of fibers and cells throughout the lymph vessels and bodily organs that contain lymphocytes; also called lymphoid tissue.

Lymphatic trunk A large vessel that drains lymph from extensive areas of the body. The intestinal lymphatic trunk drains the intestines and abdominal wall; the lumbar lymphatic trunk drain the legs, lower abdominal organs, and pelvis. The intercostal and bronchomediastinal lymphatic trunks receive lymph from portions of the thorax; the subclavian lymphatic trunk drains the arm; and the jugular lymphatic trunk receives lymph fluid from the neck and head. These trunks merge into either the thoracic duct or the right lymphatic trunk, and lymph then flows into the veins and enters the bloodstream.

Lymphatic vessel A vessel larger than a lymph capillary; the channel through which lymph flows.

Lymphedema Chronic localized fluid retention and swelling that results from venous or lymphatic vessel malformation. Primary lymphedema, also called congenital lymphedema, is swelling that results from the obstruction of lymph vessels and/or nodes due to an inborn defect. Secondary lymphedema, also called obstructive lymphedema, is caused by injury, disease or parasitic infection. Secondary lymphedema is most frequently seen after lymph node dissection, surgery, and/or radiation therapy.

Lymphocyte A white blood cell formed in lymphatic tissue (lymph nodes, spleen, thymus, tonsils, Peyer's patches, and bone marrow). The primary types are T- and B-cells, and natural killer (NK) cells.

Lymphoid Of, relating to, or referring to lymph tissue or the lymphatic system.

Lymphoscintigraphy A medical imaging study in which images of the lymphatic system are obtained with the assistance of a radioactive tracer material.

Lymphotome A specific section of the body having a network of lymph nodes that drains it. There are four main lymphotomes in the trunk of the body. See also *watersheds.*

Macrophage A white blood cell that is a mature monocyte, and digests pathogens in the bloodstream and tissues; also called a phagocyte.

Metabolic waste By-products of cellular activities that are not needed by the body and are excreted.

Monocyte An immature macrophage; a large leukocyte.

Natural killer (NK) cell A lymphocyte that destroys virus-infected cells.

Neutrophil A type of phagocytotic white blood cell that destroys microorganisms; it also migrates to the site of an injury immediately after trauma and during the acute phase of inflammation. It is the most abundant type of white blood cells in mammals.

Nonspecific immunity Resistance to disease provided by mechanical and chemical barriers to invading cells without memory for specific antigens or the creation of antibodies. Also known as innate immunity, or natural immunity.

Passive immunity Resistance to disease acquired through the transfer of antibodies from another person, usually from mother to fetus. Also known as acquired immunity.

Peyer's patches An aggregated mass of flat, oval, elevated nodules of lymph tissue containing white blood cells, located on the mucosa of the small intestine. Peyer's patches recognize antigens in food and trigger a defensive reaction to them. Also called Peyer's glands.

Phagocytes Cells that destroy microorganisms and foreign particles by absorbing and destroying them.

Phlebitis Inflammation of a vein, usually in the legs. When there is a clot causing the inflammation, the condition is called thrombophlebitis.

Pitting edema A swollen area characterized by an indentation (pit) that takes time to fill back in after pressure is applied.

Plasma The liquid constituent of blood, in which blood cells are suspended. (Distinguished from serum, which is obtained after coagulation of the fibrin and red blood cells in the plasma.)

Platelet A particle in blood that forms a clot when an injury is detected. Numerous platelets stick to each other and to damaged areas in blood vessels.

Precollector An initial lymph vessel that absorbs lymph from tissues and directs it into other lymph vessels.

Primary lymphedema A disease caused by the congenital malformation of the lymph vessels, which results in chronic swelling of a body part.

Reticular tissue Branching strands of collagen that form a lattice-like support for structures such as organs and lymph nodes. Reticular tissue is inelastic and fixed in place, but because of its open structure, fluid and cells are able to migrate through it. (Reticular means "resembling a net.")

Right lymphatic duct One of the two largest lymph vessels; receives lymph fluid from the right arm, the right side of the upper trunk, and the right side of the neck and head, and then delivers the fluid to the right subclavian vein. (Note: The left lymphatic duct is called the thoracic duct.)

Secondary lymphedema Obstruction of lymph vessels due to infection, injury, irradiation, or surgery. Also called lymphatic obstruction.

Sentinel node biopsy A medical procedure performed to determine whether breast cancer has spread to axillary (underarm) lymph nodes. A blue radioactive tracer and/or blue dye is injected into the area of the breast tumor. The lymphatic vessels carry the dye or radioactive material to the first lymph node receiving fluid from the tumor (the sentinel node), and the one most likely to contain cancer cells if the cancer has spread. Only if the sentinel node contains cancer cells are more lymph nodes removed.

Soma The body of an organism.

Specific immunity Immunity resulting from the creation of antibodies that remember and destroy microorganisms after the first exposure, and mount stronger attacks each subsequent time that the pathogen is encountered; is activated by the innate immune system. Also called adaptive immunity or acquired immunity.

Spleen A lymph organ that stores blood, and produces lymphocytes and monocytes. It is located along blood vessels rather than lymph vessels and is considered to be the "lymph node of the blood."

Stationary circle A massage movement conducted using flat fingers; the skin is gently contacted, compressed slightly, and then the tissue is stretched with a circular movement toward the lymph nodes.

T-cells Lymphocytes that attacks foreign cells; they differentiate into helper T-cells, suppressor T-cells, and natural killer (NK) T-cells. They are formed in the bone marrow and then migrate to the thymus; the T in the name stands for thymus. Also called T-lymphocytes.

Thoracic duct The main lymphatic trunk and the largest lymph vessel; it drains fluid from the lower body, viscera, upper left trunk and arm, and left side of the head and neck, and empties into the left subclavian vein.

Thymus A lymphoid organ consisting of connective tissue and lymph tissue. It produces four hormones that send the signal for B-cells and T-cells to mature. It is the organ in which T-cells mature and multiply; it provides immunity to infants and children and then atrophies upon puberty.

Tonsils Lymph nodes located on either side of the throat at the opening to the respiratory and digestive tracts. Their job is to destroy foreign cells and particles that enter those tracts; includes pharyngeal, palatine, and lingual tonsils.

Toxins Bacteria, viruses, fungi, parasites, harmful chemicals and harmful microscopic particles; can cause disease at low concentrations.

Venous angle The angle formed by the junction of the internal, external, and anterior jugular veins and the subclavian vein with the thoracic duct on the left side, or the right lymphatic duct on the right side; it occurs in the posterior cervical angle.

Watershed The line between any two lymphotomes is called a watershed. The sagittal watershed extends from the top of the head to the perineum and divides the right and left lymphtomes. The upper horizontal watershed separates the drainage pathways of the head and neck from the trunk. The horizontal watershed divides the trunk at the level of the navel and the lower margins of the ribs, separating upper and lower lymphotomes of the trunk.

Australasian Lymphology Association, AUS
PO Box 37
Mount Colah NSW 2079
Fax: 02 9847 5013
E-mail: info@lymphology.asn.au
URL: http://lymphology.asn.au/new/
index.php

Lymphoedema Support Network, UK
St. Luke's Crypt
Sydney Street
London
SW3 6NH
Telephone: 020 7351 0990
Fax: 020 7349 9809
E-mail: adminlsn@lymphoedema.
freeserve.co.uk
URL: http://www.lymphoedema.org/

Földi School, Germany
Földischule
Zum Engelberg 18
79249 Merzhausen
Telefon: +49 761 406921
Telefax: +49 761 406983
E-mail: info@foeldischule.de
URL: http://www.foeldischule.de

International Society of Lymphology, USA
Lymphology Journal
Arizona Health Sciences Center
Dept. of Surgery (GS and T)
P.O. Box 245063
Tucson AZ 85724-5063
E-mail: lymph@u.arizona.edu
URL: http://www.u.arizona.edu/~witte/
ISL.htm

Lymphedema Association of Australia, AUS
URL: http://lymphoedema.org.au

Lymphatic Research Foundation, USA
40 Garvies Point Road, Suite D
Glen Cove, NY 11542
Telephone: (516) 625-9675
Fax: (516) 625-9410
E-mail: lrf@lymphaticresearch.org
URL: www.lymphaticresearch.org/

National Lymphedema Network, USA
116 New Montgomery Street,
Suite 235
San Francisco, CA 94015
Telephone: (415) 908-3681
URL: www.lymphnet.org

Lymphology Association of North America, USA
L.A.N.A.
P.O. Box 466
Wilmette, IL 60091
USA773-756-8971
E-mail: lana@clt-lana.org
URL: www.clt-lana.org

A

abdominal massage
  contraindications for, 118–119
  muscles/fascia and, 124–135
  organs and, 122–124
  purpose of, 117–118
  structure and, 118–122
acquired immunity, 35
active immunity, 35
adenoids, 21
adipose tissue, 10–11
afferent vessels
  abdominal massage and, 127–130
  defined, 18
  face/neck treatment and, 78–80
  location, 20
  lower extremities/trunk and, 105–106
  upper extremities/trunk and, 93
aggregated lymph nodules, 22
allergies
  as contraindication for LDM, 51, 75
  edema and, 41
antigens, 19–20
aponeuroses, 11
areolar (loose) connective tissue, 10
artificial immunity, 35
Asdonk, Johannes, 2
asthma, 51
  as contraindication for LDM, 75
autoimmune diseases, 34
axilla, 21
axillary, 60–61

B

basement membrane, 16–17
basophils, 36
blood, composition/function of, 12–14
blood clot, 49–50
blood pressure
  as contraindication for LDM, 51–52
  as function of lymphatic system, 29
  lymphatic circulation and, 26
body wraps, 149–150
boundaries and emotional release, 144
breathing
  abdominal massage and, 117
  lymphatic circulation and, 25–26
  and preparation for LDM, 71
broncomediastinal trunks, 18
B-/T-lymphocytes, 36–37

C

capillaries, 16–17
cartilage, 11–12
cells and immunity, 35–37
cellulite, 150–155
cervical nodes, 61
chemical resistance and immunity, 33
chyle, 18, 30, 43

circulation
  initial lymphatics and, 24–26
  lymph drainage pathways and, 26–27
cisterna chyli, 118, 127, 135
cleanliness, 71
client
  abdominal massage and, 135
  emotional release in, 141–144
  information regarding, 52–55,
    70, 72–73
  preparation for mind-body effects,
    138–140
  relationship with therapist, 71–72
clinical setting for LDM, 3
columnar epithelial cells, 9
communication during LDM, 69
comprehensive decongestive therapy
  (CDT), 2
connective tissue
  abdominal massage and, 118,
    132–134
  cellulite and, 150–154
  composition/function of, 9–12
  lymphedema and, 5
contraindications for LDM, 49–52, 75–76,
  104, 118–119, 146, 149

D

data, 52–55, 70
dense fibrous tissue, 11
depression, 48
detoxification treatments, 148–150
diaphragm, 125
diet, 48
dietary fat, 30
direction of movement during LDM,
  59, 63–64
diseases. *See also* treatments concurrent
  with LDM
  autoimmune, 34
  as contraindication for LDM, 50, 75
  edema and, 40
  primary/secondary lymphedema, 4–5
drainage pathways, 26–27, 62, 82–83

E

edema
  defined, 2
  as indication for LDM, 46
  lymphedema disease, 41–44
  positional, 48
  understanding, 4, 39–41
efferent vessels
  abdominal massage and, 127–130
  defined, 18
  face/neck treatment and, 78–80
  lower extremities/trunk and, 105–106
  upper extremities/trunk and, 93
effleurage, 65–66

elephantiasis, 5, 43
embolism, 49–50
emotional tension
    edema and, 41
    and release, 141–144
endothelial cells, 16
energetic effects of LDM
    client preparation, 138–140
    and emotional release in clients,
        141–144
    healing crisis, 135
    healing crisis and, 140–141,
        174–175
    meditative touch for, 137–138
    proper setting for, 137
    treatment concurrent with LDM
        for, 148
enmeshment and emotional
    release, 143
eosinophils, 36
epithelial cells, 8–9
epithelial tissue, 8–9
erythrocytes, 12–13
exercise
    cellulite and, 151
    edema and, 39–40
    lymphatic circulation and, 25–26
external oblique, 124–125

F

face. *See* head massage
facilities, 3, 71, 137
fascia, 126–127
fasciae, 11
fasting, 149–150
fatigue, 48
fibrosis, 42, 58, 147–148
flap valves, 16
fluid balance, 29

G

German Society of Lymphology, 2

H

head massage
    drainage pathways, 82–83
    indications/
        contraindications, 75–76
    locating nodes, 77–81
    massage outline for head, 83–90
    massage outline for neck, 83–85
    observing/palpating nodes, 81–82
    self-massage, 158, 160–163
    swollen nodes, 76–77
healing
    as function of lymphatic
        system, 30
    microcirculation and, 3
healing crisis, 135, 140–141,
    174–175

I

identification and emotional
    release, 143
iliacus, 125–126
ilium, 120–121
immune system
    as indication for LDM, 47
    and LDM for wellness, 3
    LDM stimulation of, 2–3
immunity
    acquired, 35
    cell types and, 35–37
    as function of lymphatic system, 29
    inflammation and, 33–34
    nonspecific, 33
    specific, 34
indications for LDM, 46–49, 75–76
infectious conditions, 51
inflammation
    abdominal massage and, 117
    cellulite and, 151–152
    as contraindication for LDM, 75–76
    immunity and, 33–34
    lymphedema and, 5
intake form as record, 52–55, 70
internal oblique, 124–125
interstitial fluid, 2
intestinal trunk, 18

J

"J" stroke, 64–65
judgment and emotional release, 143
jugular trunk, 18, 78

L

lacteals, 14, 30
leukocytes, 12–13
levator ani, 126
ligaments, 11
lingual tonsils, 21
lipedema, 150
liposuction, 152
lumbar trunks, 18
lymph
    composition/function of, 15–16
    as transporter, 13
lymph circulation. *See* circulation
lymph diseases. *See also* diseases
    primary lymphedema, 4–5
    secondary lymphedema, 5
lymph drainage massage (LDM). *See
    also* energetic effects of LDM; self-
    massage
    beginning session of, 72
    communication during session, 69
    contraindications (abdominal),
        118–119
    contraindications (lower extremity/
        trunk), 104

contraindications for, 49–52
defined, 2
detailed methodology (upper
    extremities/trunk), 95–102
drainage pathways (face/neck
    treatment), 82–83
drainage patterns, 60–63
history of, 2
indications (lower extremities/
    trunk), 104
indications (upper extremities/
    trunk), 92
indications for, 46–49
indications/contraindications (face/
    neck treatment), 75–76
intake form for, 52–55
intake interview/consultation
    and, 70
    after liposuction, 152
locating nodes (face/neck
    treatment), 77–81
massage outline for head (face/neck
    treatment), 83–90
massage outline for neck (face/neck
    treatment), 83–85
movement types, 64–66
muscles/fascia (abdominal) and,
    124–135
node location (upper extremities/
    trunk), 92–95
observing/palpating nodes (face/
    neck treatment), 81–82
organs (abdominal) and, 122–124
preparation for, 70–72
principles of, 57–59
purpose (abdominal), 117–118
recording client information
    after, 72–73
sequence of, 63–64
structure (abdominal) and,
    118–122
swollen nodes (face/neck
    treatment), 76–77
understanding, 2–4
using with other treatments. *See
    treatments concurrent with LDM*
lymph nodes. *See also* lymph drainage
    massage (LDM)
    abdominal massage and, 119,
        127–132
    composition/function of, 19–21
    detailed methodology (lower
        extremities/trunk), 107–115
    drainage pathways (face/neck
        treatment), 82–83
    LDM and, 2
    locating (lower extremities/trunk),
        104–105
    locating (upper extremities/
        trunk), 92–95

locating nodes (face/neck treatment), 77–81
massage outline for head (face/neck treatment), 83–90
massage outline for neck (face/neck treatment), 83–85
observing/palpating (face/neck treatment), 81–82
observing/palpating inguinal, 106–107
quadrants and, 61–63
swollen nodes (face/neck treatment), 76–77
lymph nodules, 14
lymph organs, 21
lymph stasis, 4
lymph vessels, 8–9, 16–18
lymphangiography, 42
lymphangions, 14, 17, 25
lymphatic ducts, 16
lymphatic pump, 14
lymphatic system
functions of, 29–30
and integrated functions of organ systems, 14–15
LDM's mimicry of, 2
lymph and, 15–16
lymph nodes and, 19–21
lymph vessels and, 16–18
tonsils as lymphatic tissue, 21
tonsils/spleen/thymus (lymph organs), 21–22
lymphatic trunks, 16, 18
lymphatic vessels, 2
lymphedema disease
defined, 41–43
diagnosis of, 42
effects of, 5
primary lymphedema, 43
secondary lymphedema, 43
stages of, 44
working with, 5, 43–44
lymphocytes, 2
lymphoscintigraphy, 42
lymphotomes, 26–27

M
macrophages, 21, 36
massage sequence, 63–64
mechanical resistance and immunity, 33
medication, edema and, 40
meditative touch, 137–139
menstrual cycle, 41
metabolic waste, 12–13
mind-body effects of LDM. See energetic effects of LDM
monocytes, 34, 36
movement and lymphatic circulation, 25–26

muscle cells, 12
muscles/fascia, abdominal massage and, 124–127, 134–135
music and LDM, 70–71

N
natural killer (NK) cells, 36
neck massage
drainage pathways, 82–83
indications/contraindications, 75–76
locating nodes, 77–81
massage outline for head, 83–90
massage outline for neck, 83–85
observing/palpating nodes, 81–82
self-massage, 158–159
swollen nodes, 76–77
nerve cells, 12
neutrophils, 34, 36
nonspecific immunity, 33

O
obesity, cellulite and, 150
organ systems
lymph organs, 21–22
lymphatic system, 15–21. See also lymphatic system
organs and abdominal massage, 122–124

P
pain
intake form and, 54
LDM and, 3, 76
palatine tonsils, 21
palpation, 57–58
parasites, elephantiasis and, 5
passive immunity, 35
people-pleaser and emotional release, 143–144
phagocytes, 19–20
pharyngeal tonsils, 21
phlebitis, 49–50, 75
piriformis, 126
plasma, 13–14
platelets, 12–13
positional edema, 48
precollectors, 17–18
pregnancy, 118–119, 149
pressure application during LDM, 58–59
primary lymphedema, 4–5, 43
professionalism, 71
psoas major, 125–126
pump, 64

Q
quadrants, 61–63
quadratus lumborum, 125–126

R
radiation therapy, edema and, 40
rectus abdominis, 124–125
relaxation, 2–3
research
importance of staying current, 4
and lymphatic system regeneration, 30
reticular tissue, 10
rhythm/repetition during LDM, 59
ribs, 120
right lymphatic duct, 18–19

S
salt, 40
scar tissue
abdominal massage and, 117
edema and, 40
as indication for LDM, 48–49
inflammation and, 5
LDM and, 3
lymphedema disease and, 42–43
treatment concurrent with LDM for, 147–148
secondary lymphedema, 5, 43
self-massage
face, 158, 160–163
lower limbs, 169–171
neck, 158–159
reasons for, 157
soft-tissue injury and, 172
upper limbs, 164–168
skeletal structure, 119–122
skin care, 148
skin enhancement, 49
skin movement during LDM, 58
smooth (nonstriated involuntary) muscle tissue, 12
soft tissue injury, 47–48, 146–147, 172
specific immunity, 34
spine, 120
spleen, 10, 21
splinting, 34
squamous epithelial cells, 9
stationary circle, 64
stress
edema and, 41
as indication for LDM, 47–48
surgery, as indication for LDM, 47

T
T-/B-lymphocytes, 36–37
T-cells, 22
tendons, 11, 117
thrombosis, 49–50, 75
thymus, 14, 21–22
thyroid problems, 51, 75

tissues
    blood/lymph and, 12–14
    connective, 9–12
    epithelial, 8–9
    muscle cells and, 12
    nerve cells and, 12
    protein buildup prevention
        in, 29–30
tonsils, 21
toxins
    body wraps and, 149–150

    and lymph as transporter, 14, 76
    microcirculation and, 3
transversus abdominis, 124–125
treatments concurrent with LDM
    body-mind therapies, 148
    cellulite and, 150–155
    complementing skin care, 148
    detoxification treatments and,
        148–150
    fibrosis/scar tissue and, 147–148
    soft-tissue injury and, 146–147

V
venous angle, 16
Vodder, Emil, 2–3
von Winiwater, Alexander, 2

W
watersheds, 27, 60–62
wellness setting for LDM, 3

CPSIA information can be obtained
at www.ICGtesting.com
Printed in the USA
FFOW03n0553190117
31522FF